DID YOU KNOW . . .

- High levels of blood sugar can prematurely age your organs?

- Many prescription and over-the-counter drugs generate free radicals, substances which greatly contribute to the aging process?

- Vitamin E works almost as well as the blood-thinning drug warfarin (Coumadin) and has also shown promise in enhancing memory?

- Contrary to popular belief, eating eggs actually improves your blood cholesterol profile?

- Melatonin, widely known as a sleep supplement, also has effective antioxidant properties?

DISCOVER MORE ESSENTIAL ANTI-AGING FACTS IN

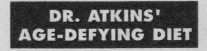

DR. ATKINS' AGE-DEFYING DIET

Also by Robert C. Atkins, M.D.

Dr. Atkins' New Diet Revolution
Dr. Atkins' Vita-Nutrient Solution
Dr. Atkins' Quick and Easy New Diet Cookbook
Dr. Atkins' Diet Revolution
Dr. Atkins' Health Revolution
Dr. Atkins' Nutrition Breakthrough
Dr. Atkins' Super Energy Diet

DR. ATKINS' AGE-DEFYING DIET

Robert C. Atkins, M.D.

with Sheila Buff

St. Martin's Paperbacks

DR. ATKINS' AGE-DEFYING DIET

Copyright © 2001 by Robert C. Atkins.

Cover photograph by © Hilmar.

ISBN: 0-312-97701-8

Printed in the United States of America

St. Martin's Paperbacks edition / January 2001

St. Martin's Paperbacks are published by St. Martin's Press, 175 Fifth Avenue, New York, N.Y. 10010.

20 19 18 17 16 15 14 13

*To my many activist followers,
who are determined to spread
the truths that will make
the world a healthier place*

CONTENTS

NOTE TO THE READER

The information offered in this book, although based on the author's experience with many thousands of patients, is not intended to be a substitute for the advice and counsel of your personal physician. While the recommendations are appropriate for most people, each individual may have different requirements based on a full medical profile. No one regime fits all.

1

A PROGRAM FOR DEFYING AGING

What if you could grow old without feeling the effects of age, without succumbing to the physical and mental decline assumed to be the inevitable companion to aging?

You can. The decline is not inevitable. On the contrary. It is possible to look and feel good, both physically and mentally, throughout a very long life.

How do I know? I've been a full-time medical practitioner for more than forty years, and in that time, the Atkins Center in New York City has treated more than 65,000 patients. A great many of these have been elderly patients suffering from all those degenerative ailments we associate with being old: osteoporosis, failing eyesight, senility, heart disease, diabetes. By defying the conventional wisdom, and by applying many of the medical innovations that conventional wisdom disdains, the Atkins Center has brought new life to the vast majority of these elderly patients. They have become younger—not chronologically, since no one can literally turn back time—but by all the usual medical measures. This means that their laboratory results and all the measures of their physical and mental capacities are better than they were when the patients first came to the Center. It also means that the rate at which these patients encounter the problems attributed to aging have slowed, often to a remarkable degree.

Right now, at the start of the twenty-first century, the know-how for defying the effects of aging is in our hands. The scientific breakthroughs come at us with startling rapidity. The evidence is there—even if the medical mainstream stubbornly dismisses the evidence, or ignores it, or insists that more study is needed to make absolutely sure.

Most of what we call aging is simply the presence of disease—chronic, ubiquitous disease that undermines our body so consistently that we universally accept the deterioration as the consequence of "getting older." Nothing could be farther from the truth. Many of these common ailments can be prevented or reduced.

What causes these ailments? What sets in motion the processes of aging? We'll look closely at the characteristics and underlying causes of the so-called diseases of aging in the chapters that follow. We'll see that there are very specific reasons why certain aging diseases— cardiovascular ailments and diabetes in particular— became so common in the latter part of the twentieth century, and why they were not common before. We'll see just how the aging factors of these diseases work.

Once we know why we suffer these ailments and what the underlying causes are, it's possible to create a strategy to fight back, a program to defy the effects of aging, no matter how old we become.

FIRST, DEFY PREVAILING BELIEFS

There's a lot more you *could* know about defying aging than you're being told.

Evidence about ways to live healthier and longer lives is too often caught in the crosscurrents of modern science. While the currents of scientific discovery provide the breakthrough information we need to defy the effects of aging, the crosscurrents of economic self-interest preserve the status quo and prevents those breakthroughs from getting the widespread use and acceptance they deserve.

In the area of nutrition, for example, the potential of vitamins and minerals to fight disease and defy age is a case in point. It wasn't until 1920 that vitamins were identified; over the next eighty years, more and more nutritional substances were discovered, as were their roles and functions in preserving and restoring health. By now, thousands of scientific studies have been performed showing that such substances are often better and safer than drugs in overcoming and preventing illness. But the medical community, which by the early 1900s was already single-mindedly devoted to a pharmaceuticals-only treatment system, found no place for these substances in its consensus protocols. Vitamins and minerals were banished from the disease-fighting curriculum at medical schools, and remain so, with rare exceptions, to this day.

Nature's herbs offer another example. Their medicinal use dates back many centuries, but the scientific analysis of why and how they accomplished their healing was done only in recent years. And the analysis offers compelling evidence for the power of many herbs to slow or reverse the effects of aging. But again, no place was found for their benefits in the medical mainstream.

Caught in the same crosscurrent are such discoveries as hormonal balancing, probiotic bacterial balancing, chelation therapy, detoxification, and more age-defying techniques presented later in this book. All have achieved support in various scientific studies but none are in common usage.

That leaves us today with a unique opportunity for major health progress. As the nutritional breakthroughs continue to pour forth from the laboratories, all you need is an awareness of when going along with the system will help you defy age, and when defying the system helps get you to your goal—as you take advantage of the knowledge that courageous, innovative scientists have already provided us.

The age-defying program in this book provides that awareness. It embraces *what works*—a range of techniques and practices and nutritional advice to defy the effects of aging, whether the knowledge comes from those who cling to prevailing beliefs or from defying prevailing beliefs. For those of us who don't have much time to waste, the program in this book frees scientific discovery from the eddy of scientific policy-making and puts the evidence where it belongs—right in our hands.

A TWO-PRONGED ATTACK

There are basically two ways to defy age. One is by using techniques so health-promoting they seem to turn back the clock. When you are healthier overall, you are better equipped to defy the disease processes associated with aging, to stop them before they have a chance to begin. The other way to defy age is by reversing the disease processes that may be present, especially cardiovascular disease, the scourge of our era.

The program I present in this book does both.

The key to both is diet. Whether reversing a disease process that has already taken hold or equipping yourself to fight off incipient ailments, diet can be a formidable weapon. I use the word "diet" loosely. After all, I have something of a reputation as the author of an effective weight-loss diet. But this book is not aimed at showing you how to lose weight the luxurious Atkins way, although it will certainly help you do so if you need to. Rather, the Age-Defying Diet is an overall nutritional plan aimed at eliminating the aging factors from your life now while optimizing your body's ability to fight them off in the future.

But diet isn't enough. In recent years, there have been many discoveries about the important role of vitamins, minerals, amino acids, fatty acids, herbs, hormones, and other forms of natural nourishment. I call these substances vitanutrients—*vita* is the Latin word for "life," of course, and vitanutrients truly nourish and sustain life. Where pharmaceutical drugs actually inhibit normal body processes, vitanutrients are enablers that facilitate the body's natural physiology. They are also generally safe, effective, and typically inexpensive remedies that can replace the drugs and invasive procedures that enrich the mainstream medical establishment, which could be why the mainstream medical establishment tends to dismiss vitanutrients as unimportant. The evidence, however, as I'll discuss later in the book, demonstrates that supplementing your diet with vitanutrients can be tremendously important in eliminating many of the ailments of aging.

So can exercise, of course. You've heard that before, but the program in this book will show you specifically how and why exercise defeats aging.

My Age-Defying Diet combines all three of these age-opposing weapons—diet, supplemental nutrition, and exercise. I'll teach you what specific combinations to use to clean out the toxins from your body, rejuvenate aging organs, counteract adverse environmental impacts, restore healthy bacteria to your digestive tract, optimize your brain power, and much more. The tools for doing the job are all right here, easily available and demonstrably effective. The "authorities" may not tell you so, but authority should always be questioned.

Are you getting older? Then you know it's time for a revolution. It starts now.

2

THE AGING DISEASES OF OUR TIME AND PLACE

We're not dying the way we used to. A century ago, older people—and often the very young—were routinely swept to premature deaths by an array of infectious disease.

But those diseases are a thing of the past. Influenza epidemics, smallpox, tuberculosis, and polio have all been virtually wiped off the face of the earth (despite some recent recurrences) by the scientific discoveries of the twentieth century. In my view, these discoveries represent the greatest compilation of life-extending breakthroughs ever achieved. No other century—no other *five centuries*, I would wager—could equal the impact on life span of the twentieth century, in which science gained control over infectious disease and eliminated the major causes of premature death that had plagued mankind for millennia.

There's plenty of credit to go around for this achievement—to scientists in the lab, to public health officials who worked to control disease transmission, to surgeons who developed hundreds of procedures that successfully converted life-threatening illnesses into momentary nuisances.

The magnitude of the achievement is easily defined: We started the twentieth century with a collective life expectancy of 45 years; at last count, life expectancy had expanded to 76.5 years on average.[1] Before 1900, 75 percent of all Americans died before age 65; today, more than 70 percent of us will live to be over 70. Improving human life expectancy so profoundly in a single century is surely a singular achievement.

But the twentieth century has a lot to answer for as well. Even as the previous century's life-shortening illnesses were conquered, new illnesses came along to keep us from achieving the goal of truly extending *healthy* life. Heart disease, diabetes, hypertension, cancer, Alzheimer's disease, and other maladies to all intents and purposes originated, or at least achieved epidemic proportions, in the twentieth century—and they're becoming even more widespread in the twenty-first. Objective observers rightly note that while we have made progress in overcoming infectious diseases and other conditions that strike us down before our time, older people still reach senility at approximately the same age.

What happened? What are we doing now that our great-grandparents did not do a century ago? Or what are we not doing that they did? What is the significant characteristic of our highly industrialized, technologically advanced Western culture that's resulting in these particular ailments? Ironically, the twentieth century produced not just the ailments but also the clue to what causes them *and* the scientific discoveries that can lead the way to their eradication.

THE "WESTERNIZATION" OF DISEASE

The big clue to the nature of our current diseases has been known since at least 1974. That's when a brilliant physician named T. L. Cleave, a surgeon-captain in Britain's Royal Navy and a former director of medical research at the Institute of Naval Medicine, published an epidemiological study called *The Saccharine Disease*. This work, now unfortunately out of print, has long had my vote for the number-one health book of the twentieth century.

Cleave made a careful study of hospital records of Third World nations, mainly in Africa, and observed that virtually no single native ever suffered obesity, diabetes, colon cancer, gallstones, diverticulitis, or heart disease. These diseases, the common illnesses of advanced Western cultures, were not simply less frequent in the places Cleave studied; they were nonexistent.

Clearly, as Cleave saw, the overriding point of differentiation between the cultures he was studying and the Western culture from which he came was diet. Cleave concluded, therefore, that the "Western" twentieth-century diseases were diet-related disorders. But that was only part of his conclusion.

Unlike his colleague Dr. Dennis Burkitt, who looked at the same type of data and concluded that the high dietary fiber these people ate was what protected them, Cleave was convinced that it was the other side of the coin that did the trick. In his view—and in mine—the absence of refined carbohydrates in the diets protected the Third World peoples from the array of twentieth-century illnesses so prevalent on our side of the cultural divide.

THE RULE OF TWENTY YEARS

Cleave went further. He suggested that within twenty years of refined-carbohydrate foods being introduced into the native diet and replacing the indigenous foods, diabetes and heart disease would begin to appear in the population. Within forty years, he said, these diseases would be widespread. Cleave dubbed this his Rule of Twenty Years, and I've seen it proven time and again.

Item: Both diabetes and coronary heart attack deaths began to appear in Iceland twenty years after sugar was made a major dietary component.[2]

Item: Among Yemenite Jews living a traditional life in Yemen, diabetes had been virtually unknown. In 1977, about twenty-five years after these nomadic Jews moved to Israel and gave up their traditional unrefined carbohydrate diet in favor of a more Westernized diet that was high in sugar, Israeli studies showed that their rate of diabetes and glucose intolerance reached 11.8 percent.[3] And—coronary heart disease began to appear among them!

Item: In Saudi Arabia, diabetes and associated heart disease have emerged almost exactly twenty years after refined carbohydrates and a more Westernized diet became the norm. Today in Saudi Arabia, diabetes afflicts 12 percent of the men who live in urban areas and 14 percent of the women. Among urban women age fifty-one to sixty, the prevalence of diabetes is an astonishing 49 percent. In the rural populations, where people still retain remnants of their traditional diet, the rates are lower but still high: 7 percent for men and 7.7 percent for women. Saudi Arabia has gone from being a country that had virtually no diabetes before 1970 to having one of the highest rates of diabetes in the world.[4]

Cleave was right on target, and his Rule of Twenty Years is also proving true in Japan, India, Mexico, and many other countries. Its greatest value, in my opinion, lies in its prophetic power: It can predict when epidemic increases in diabetes, diabetes-induced heart disease, and a range of related conditions will take place.

THE DIET DISTINCTION

But the rule also helps us answer a lot of nagging questions: Why was cardiology a minor specialty in Japan in the 1950s but a major necessity now? Why is Asia the new hotbed of a diabetes epidemic exceeding 100 million cases? Why does the World Health Organization project a 170 percent growth in the number of people with diabetes in developing countries by 2025, from 84 million people to 228 million people? Why is the worldwide rise in diabetes projected to be 122 percent, from 135 million people to 300 million? Why will diabetes nearly double in India between 1995 and 2025?

The answer to all these questions is the same: The rise in these particular diseases is the consequence of the Westernization of these cultures, which in biologic terms means the dietary acceptance of refined carbohydrates. Cleave's discoveries thus constitute a large part of the basis for understanding the incidence of modern illness in all parts of the world.

The discoveries may also have been before their time. That is, the phenomenon was observed before the scientific explanation was worked out. But all that is water under the bridge. So much evidence has since been amassed linking refined carbohydrates to sugar and insulin disorders, and these disorders to heart disease, hypertension, and stroke, that any medical advisory board member entrusted with making public health policy who remains silent on this matter must, in my view, be deemed guilty of malfeasance. In plainer language, this means that members of the medical establishment who continue to recommend sugar-laden cereals as heart-healthy should perhaps be consulting with their defense attorneys.

Heart disease, as is well known, is the number-one cause of death and of shortened life span in Western culture. Heart disease achieved that dubious distinction, in large part, because of errors of judgment on the part of the health powers-that-be and because of their stubborn refusal to correct those errors. In my opinion, those errors of judgment in essence created and perpetuated the majority of life-threatening and life-shortening diseases that today provide the greatest deterrent to our reaching our full life spans.

Yet the twentieth century ended with the scientific know-how to eradicate those diseases. The scientific avant-garde did its job well; the fruits of their collective labor show clearly the diet-related component of these diseases. Only the political and economic know-how still eludes us, not the scientific know-how. That's why it's important to look at the whole issue of diet-related disorders more closely, and there's no better target for our exploration than our number-one killer—heart disease.

3

THE HEART OF THE MATTER

Atherosclerosis. The word comes from two Greek words: *athero*, which means "gruel" or "paste," and *sclerosis*, which means "hardness." In atherosclerosis, a kind of gruel made up of fatty deposits, cholesterol, cellular waste products, and other substances builds up in the inner lining of an artery. The buildup then hardens. This is known as plaque, and it eventually will partially or totally block the flow of blood through the artery.

Atherosclerosis is the quintessential ailment of the twentieth century—and now of the twenty-first century. Eradicate it and scientists have estimated we will extend our collective life expectancy by six, eight, even a dozen years. They would be healthy years, unmarred by chronic illness and disability, by the limitations on our activity and the signs of aging that result from narrowed, poorly functioning blood vessels.

Can we eradicate it? Yes. To find out how, we just need to go back in time a bit, for ironically, atherosclerotic cardiovascular disease, the major illness associated with age, was virtually unheard of a century ago. In that case, shouldn't it be possible to figure out the precise conditions that have brought about this epidemic? Certainly. In fact, it's been "figured out" for some time. Why, then, hasn't the disease been eradicated?

The answer to that is a little tougher. For I'll wager it will take a good deal of convincing to bring you to the conclusion I reached decades ago, a conclusion that has allowed me to reverse the time clock on thousands of my patients. It is this: People have been lied to about heart disease for so long that even scholarly researchers without a dishonest bone in their bodies are repeating these whoppers without a smidgen of suspicion that they could be untrue.

So before we learn how heart disease can be slowed and actually reversed, it's essential to unlearn the received "wisdom" the medical establishment keeps feeding us. And that means finding out the truth about what I call The Gospel According to the American Heart Association.

AN EXPENSIVE FICTION

The truth is that the heart-health message fostered over the years by the medical establishment is a fiction—an expensive fiction if you count up the costs of the research that still *cannot prove the message*, and a very expensive fiction when you add in the human costs in disease and shortened life span. The fiction starts with bad science and ends in bad advice to the public. In my view, it's an advanced fiction, one fueled by economic interests that should not be calling the tune for the nation's health. Once we understand the fiction, we can disenthrall ourselves of it and move on to discover the real causes of aging diseases and effective ways to defy aging.

The Gospel According to the AHA is repeated in similar form by the American Medical Association, the American Dietetic Association, the U.S. government, and the National Cholesterol Education Program. All of them agree unquestioningly that for an individual to achieve heart health, the following articles of faith must be adhered to:

- All dietary fats must be restricted, especially saturated fats.
- Dietary cholesterol must be nearly eliminated.
- Margarine and other polyunsaturated fats are healthier than butter and other saturated fats and should replace them.
- Carbohydrates made with white flour should be the basis of a healthy diet.
- Eating ten teaspoons of sugar a day is perfectly healthy.

New scientific information from even the most prestigious journals that counters any of these articles of faith is simply not heeded by the medical establishment. Recent studies, for example, pointing clearly to the deleterious effects of trans fats—the partially hydrogenated oils used extensively in processed food and the stuff that gives margarine its buttery look—received little attention. Studies showing the heart harm that can be caused by refined junk carbohydrates made with sugar and white flour went virtually unnoticed. There has to be a reason for the medical establishment's obstinate refusal even to consider evidence that calls into question the line they've been feeding us all these years. I suggest that the reason is economic—specifically, the economic interdependence of the medical profession and the food-processing industry.

Nowhere is this mutual backslapping so well illustrated as in the American Heart Association's "Heart-Check" seal of approval on high-sugar, empty-calorie foods. You can see the Heart-Check symbol on all sorts of worthless foods, including breakfast cereals like Count Chocula and Froot Loops and such snacks as low-fat Pop-Tarts. These foods are often nothing but refined carbohydrates and may be as much as 50 percent sugar, but they have fewer than 3 grams of fat per serving, so the AHA says they're okay. The AHA's unmistakable message: Avoid fats, and nothing else matters. I hear another message behind that one: Support us enough and we'll endorse your low-fat food, no matter how fundamentally unhealthy it is.

No wonder the overwhelming majority of nutritionally concerned citizens believe in these low-fat guidelines and live by them, secure in the belief that forty years of scientific studies have proven this point beyond any doubt.

Here's *my* message: Nothing could be further from the truth. That conclusion became inescapable to me when I revamped the diet and nutritional intake of my patients and saw their illnesses dramatically reverse themselves—often disappear entirely.

But you don't have to take my word for it. The fact is that the billion-dollar research to support the hypothesis that dietary fat leads to heart disease has, with remarkable consistency, arrived at an entirely opposite result. Time and again, the research itself has proven the low-fat strategy to be a failure. Time and again, it has called the whole diet-heart hypothesis into question.

The facts speak for themselves. Here's a very well-documented fact: Heart attacks were so rare at the start of the twentieth century that the first case was not described until 1912. In 1930, heart attacks caused no more than 3,000 deaths in the United States.[1]

Based on this figure, it behooves us to ask what Americans were consuming in the early part of the century. The amount of fat in the daily diet during those first three decades of the century was somewhat greater than it is today, when we are in the midst of an epidemic of heart attacks. The three main fats our forebears ate in 1900 were lard, butter, and tallow, the hard fat obtained from beef cattle. According to today's medical establishment, both the amount and the nature of the fat consumed by those folks back in the early part of the century should have littered the streets with their corpses, as one after another they succumbed to myocardial infarction. But they didn't succumb. Their doctors had never seen a heart attack patient.

Don't these facts demand an explanation? You'll never get it from the AHA, so I guess it's up to me to explain why today's official dietary recommendations are dangerous to your health. Let's start with a closer look at the history of the diet-heart hypothesis.

DIET AND YOUR HEART: A BRIEF HISTORY

Ancel Keys was the famed nutritional researcher selected to determine the nutritional needs of GIs and design portable meals to meet those needs. He's the "K" in K rations. (Whether he was also responsible for the decision to include a cigarette with every K ration pack, I couldn't say.)

With the war over, however, Keys turned his attention to what he called the Seven Countries study, a review of diet and health around the world. The results, revealed in the early 1950s, supposedly showed that people in countries where the diet was high in saturated fat had higher rates of heart disease. Here's the fallacy: The WHO figures available to Keys totalled those of twenty nations. Keys selected the seven that proved his point.

Had he chosen other nations, fat would have been exonerated. Unfortunately, Keys' reputation was so great that the medical establishment immediately embraced his conclusions.

Based on the Keys Seven Countries study and others, equally flawed, the AHA undertook a campaign to replace butter, lard, eggs, and beef with corn oil, margarine, and cereal. By 1956, the campaign was in full swing. "Beware saturated fats" was the party line, and the medical establishment fell into place reciting it—with one notable exception. Dr. Paul Dudley White, Harvard's leading cardiologist and President Dwight Eisenhower's physician, pointed out that he hadn't seen a single coronary at Harvard between 1921 and 1928. On a televised panel discussion with other leading physicians, White proclaimed that "back in the myocardial-infarction-free days before 1920, the fats were butter and lard, and I think we would all benefit from that kind of diet." His sensible advice, based on years of clinical experience and not on epidemiological studies, was ignored.

A decade later, despite the fact that there was still no real proof of the diet-heart hypothesis, the manufacturers of Mazola corn oil and margarine nevertheless distributed a book advising us all to embrace the hypothesis and live by it. In the book, Dr. Jeremiah Stamler, one of the AHA's ringleaders, affirmed that the diet-heart theory was "enough to call for altering some habits even before the final proof is nailed down."

In an effort to find that elusive proof, Dr. Norman Jolliffe developed what he called the Prudent Diet and recruited a bunch of middle-aged businessmen to try it. The diet emphasized corn oil, margarine, and cereal. Jolliffe's control group stuck to meat, potatoes, and butter. The results? There were eight deaths from heart disease in the Prudent Diet group versus none in the meat-and-potatoes group.

Even so, the diet-heart hypothesis was already so firmly entrenched that it couldn't be uprooted. Agribusiness had far too much invested in vegetable oils, corn, wheat, and highly profitable processed foods to allow any opposition—and it had the money and government clout to bulldoze its opponents. The food industry combined with the medical establishment in strenuous efforts to suppress dissenting opinions. And dissenting opinions there were—from such eminent scientists as Dr. Fred Kummerow, Dr. Mary Enig, and Dr. George V. Mann.* The low-carbohydrate diet I published in 1973 came in for its own unscientific and totally unwarranted attack, an attack now recognizable as standard operating procedure from the medical-agribusiness establishment.

Since the Prudent Diet had not proved the point, the powers-that-be next called upon the ongoing Framingham Heart Study to do so. According to the early results of the study, those with higher total cholesterol levels had slightly more "heart events." This did not exactly confirm a connection between saturated fat in the diet and high total cholesterol. In fact, in 1992 the study's original director, Dr. William Castelli, revealed the inside story on Framingham, pointing out that the people with lowest serum cholesterol were the ones who ate the most saturated fat and cholesterol and took in the most calories.[2]

With Framingham not exactly clinching the deal,

---

*Dr. Fred Kummerow is a professor at the University of Illinois; Dr. Mary Enig is director of the Nutritional Sciences Division of Enig Associates, Inc., a fellow of the American College of Nutrition, and consulting editor of *Journal of the American College of Nutrition*; Dr. George V. Mann is a professor at Vanderbilt University.

more billions were invested to conduct and publish international studies to prove that cereal, corn oil, and margarine were heart-healthy and that most of us were candidates for cholesterol-lowering drugs. The clear aim was to ensure that the diet-heart hypothesis gained acceptance.

And gain acceptance it did—so well that it is still widely accepted today. As an ultimate badge of authenticity, the diet-heart advocates cite the 6 percent drop in death rates from cardiovascular disease between 1950 and 2000; the decline comes, the diet-heart hypothesizers say, from limiting fat in the diet.

It is certainly true that in 1950, the death rate from heart disease was 307.4 per 100,000 people, and that it went down to 134.6 per 100,000 people by 1996.[3] The overall decrease in the number of coronary episodes over the past fifty years is wonderful news, but it has one glaring shortcoming from the diet-heart point of view: Almost all of the decrease can be attributed to the significant decline in cigarette smoking (42 percent of all adults smoked in 1970), better control of blood pressure, and improved treatments for heart attack. Putting the nation on a low-fat diet—an effort that has been notably unsuccessful—has had very little to do with our declining death rate from heart attacks.

Besides, the decline in death rate is only part of the picture. Although many more of us are being saved from that first potentially fatal heart attack, we're experiencing an epidemic of heart failure instead. The reason is simple: A myocardial infarction damages and weakens the heart, which gradually works less and less efficiently.

In many cases, such heart failure is the delayed result of being treated for a first heart event by conventional doctors with cholesterol-lowering statin drugs. These drugs actually block the body's ability to produce an essential substance for producing energy in your cells, especially your heart cells. This substance is called co-enzyme Q_{10}; a shortage of it is almost certain to make a weakened heart grow weaker and eventually fail, as I'll discuss in greater detail in Chapter 9.

Whatever the particular cause, the number of heart failure patients nearly doubled in the ten years from 1989 to 1999.[4] So even though you're more likely to survive a heart attack today than you would have been fifty years ago, your chances of still being alive five years later have hardly budged over the past twenty years. Some 24 percent of men and 42 percent of women will die within one year of having a myocardial infarction; within six years of a first heart attack, 21 percent of men and 33 percent of women will have another; 7 percent of men and women will experience sudden death, and 21 percent of men and 30 percent of women will be disabled with heart failure.[5] And even with the declining death rate from heart attacks, your lifetime risk of developing heart disease is still one in two for men and one in three for women.[6]

Does this sound as if we've conquered the scourge of heart disease? Hardly. Could it be that the unholy alliance among the American Heart Association, American Medical Association, American Diabetes Association, and the U.S. government in its many manifestations has it wrong about saturated fats and the heart-diet hypothesis? It is a possibility the medical establishment seems disinclined to consider, despite the evidence that is supposed to be any scientist's guiding light.

Exacerbating the misinformation, tunnel vision, and bad science the medical establishment offers us is their number-one corollary to the heart-diet hypothesis: the belief that "one diet fits all."

It's a belief that simply flies in the face of common

sense, not to mention that it demeans the intellectual rigor we have a right to expect from our scientific leadership. Do you believe that each and every one of us should be following the same diet? Fat people and thin ones, young and old, diabetics and heart patients, Jack Spratt and his wife—should they all be eating exactly the same foods? If it's as hard for you to accept as it is for me, then you no doubt see the one-diet-fits-all belief as another fallacy to be rejected, especially when you consider the unspoken promise that the one diet contains all the nutrients anyone needs.

Bad science and bad advice. We deserve better from the medical establishment. Maybe now you see why I say that defying aging begins with defying the conventional misteachings. To understand how you too can learn to defy aging, you'll first need to understand why we age at all. That's what I'll explain next.

4

IT'S IN THE BLOOD: NUTRITION AND HEART DISEASE

In the year 1900, well before heart disease had become a leading cause of death, Americans consumed considerably more carbohydrates than they do now. Only a relatively small portion of those carbohydrates, however, could be classified as refined. Back then, grains were not milled into nutritional nothingness. And while people consumed vast quantities of sugar, it was often in the form of unrefined molasses, a rich source of iron and B vitamins. Most important, the fats our forebears ate were chiefly butter and lard; the trans fats that pump up our processed foods hadn't been invented yet. Atherosclerosis hadn't been invented yet, either—that is, it was not common, and it wasn't what aged people.

A century later, Americans consume nearly a pound a day of sugar, corn syrup, and refined grains. We eat large amounts of partially hydrogenated vegetable oils. And heart disease has become a killer of epidemic proportions.

Don't you think the American heart disease epidemic is simply another example of Cleave's theory on the linkage between nutrition and disease? Especially when you consider that my patients, by changing their nutrition to a low-carbohydrate diet, have reversed or reduced the heart disease–related aspects of the aging process?

Clearly, there's nothing "normal" about atherosclerosis at all. That's exactly why fighting off atherosclerosis presents the window of greatest opportunity to make real inroads in reversing the aging process. All we have to do is wipe out an illness that humans didn't even get until four generations ago.

To do that, we must first understand just what the illness is and what causes it. The answers are in the blood.

WHAT CAUSES A HEART ATTACK?

A heart attack is the culmination of a long process in which the arteries that feed blood to your heart and other organs gradually become blocked. Eventually, or in its most dramatic form, the blockage obstructs blood flow in one of the major arteries that supply the heart, and the result is a myocardial infarction—a heart attack.

What causes the blockage in the first place? There is no single cause. Quite reasonably, then, no single program can prevent it. The best you can do is discover what might make you uniquely vulnerable to heart problems, based on your own personal risk factors.

To start with, that means getting a complete evaluation of your blood to determine all possible risk factors for heart disease. Lab test results by themselves are not very useful until they are analyzed by a doctor who recognizes that there are many paths to heart disease. Far too many physicians today still look only at your cholesterol figures and don't even bother to test for anything else.

And that can be very misleading. Your total cholesterol figure is essentially the sum of two figures: one good, the high-density or HDL cholesterol, and one bad, the low-density or LDL cholesterol. You want the HDL to be as high as possible and the LDL to be as low as possible. So it isn't the total number that counts; it's the ratio.

A complete blood evaluation, therefore, should start with a full lipid profile—looking at the amounts of different kinds of fats in your blood—not just cholesterol but also triglycerides, very low-density lipoproteins (VLDL), and lipoprotein(a), abbreviated as Lp(a). Each of these lipid profile measures tells us something different—and all tell us something important.

YOUR LIPID PROFILE

Cholesterol is a fat-like alcohol your body needs for making sex and adrenal hormones, cell walls, and nerve sheaths. About 85 percent of the cholesterol in your body is made in your liver and in the cells of your small intestine; the rest comes from your diet.

Cholesterol is waxy, which means it's not soluble in water. To carry cholesterol around in your bloodstream, which is mostly water, your body coats it with protein; these protein-bearing cholesterol particles are called lipoproteins—*lipos* is Greek for "fat." The more protein a cholesterol particle carries, the denser it is. About 65 percent of the circulating lipoprotein in your blood is low-density lipoprotein. LDLs carry cholesterol to your cells and are the bad cholesterol. About 20 percent of your circulating lipoproteins is high-density lipoprotein. These smaller, denser cholesterol particles pick up cholesterol from your cells and carry it back to the liver for further processing; they are the good cholesterol.

Triglycerides are risk factors quite apart from cholesterol. They are very small, light fat particles that have only a tiny bit of protein attached to them. Your body sends some of your triglycerides to your muscles for energy but stores most of it as body fat.

Triglycerides are made in the liver, where they are converted into very low-density lipoproteins. VLDL may well be the lurking villain of the blood lipids. Your VLDL level goes up along with your triglyceride level and may be just as dangerous, in part because these particles get denser as they circulate in your blood until they turn into LDL cholesterol.

Lipoprotein(a), another type of cholesterol particle, seems to be most important for repairing your blood vessels. We now know that high levels of Lp(a) are predictive of heart disease, but not for the same reasons the other lipoproteins are, as I'll explain in more detail in the pages that follow.

But for now, let's examine what the lipid profile tells us about heart disease and nutrition.

HDL: THE GOOD CHOLESTEROL

For decades, mainstream cardiologists have recognized the beneficial role played by the HDL cholesterol fraction. Every ratio indicating risk of heart disease uses it as the divisor. Whether it's total cholesterol, LDL, LDL plus VLDL, or the dramatically important triglycerides, all are divided by the HDL, and it's when that number rises that your doctor feels the greatest concern. Conclusion: HDL is one number you want to be as high as possible.

How can you get it high and keep it there? It's not with a low-fat diet—quite the contrary. HDL is *lowered* by a low-fat diet, not so much by the absence of fat but by the increased consumption of carbohydrates that accompanies fat restriction. For the desired high HDL, therefore, a low-carbohydrate diet should be the rule.

TRIGLYCERIDES

Today's overemphasis on cholesterol as the sole cause of heart disease means that your doctor probably hasn't paid much attention to your triglyceride level unless it's abnormally high.

You could pay for your doctor's inattention with your life. Long ignored, high triglycerides have been convincingly shown to be an independent risk factor for heart disease—as much a risk factor as obesity, smoking, or high blood pressure.[1] Simply put, the higher your triglycerides, the greater your chance of a heart attack. This is particularly the case if you're a woman; one study estimated that 75 percent of all heart attacks in women are associated with triglyceride elevations.[2] (Another very important reason for women to lower their triglycerides is that high triglyceride levels mean a 70 percent higher risk of breast cancer. The high triglycerides seem to trigger a rise in levels of circulating estrogen, which is a significant risk factor for breast cancer.[3])

What makes triglycerides so dangerous to your heart? In large amounts, they thicken your blood and keep it from flowing easily through your blood vessels. When blood that should flow like water turns sludgy from too many triglycerides, it forms clots and can clog your blood vessels. The result is a blockage in the arteries feeding your heart—in short, a heart attack.

Most conventional doctors follow the misinformation they were taught in medical school and tell you that triglyceride levels of 250 to 500 mg/dL are perfectly normal. They're wrong, and their ignorance could be fatal to their patients. Even 200 mg/dL is too high. You need to worry about your heart health when your triglycerides are above 100 mg/dL. Above 100 mg/dL, you have twice the risk of suffering a fatal attack as someone whose level is below 100 mg/dL.[4]

HIGH TG/LOW HDL: A DEADLY COMBINATION

A high level of triglycerides is bad enough, but the combination of high triglycerides and low HDL cholesterol can be deadly, dramatically raising your risk of a heart attack. In a multiyear study of men in Muenster, Germany, in the 1980s, although only 4 percent of the study subjects had the high triglyceride/low HDL combination, 25 percent of the heart attacks occurred among men in this group.[5]

We learned why in 1997, in a study conducted at Harvard by Dr. Michael Gaziano and his colleagues that showed just how predictive of heart disease a high triglyceride/low HDL ratio really is. In the Harvard study, the participants were divided into four subgroups, or quartiles, according to ratios of triglyceride to HDL: highest, high middle, low middle, and lowest. The quartile with the highest ratio had sixteen times the likelihood of heart attacks as the lowest quartile.[6] The significance of such numbers is staggering. *No ratio has ever come close to being so predictive of heart disease.* If you are in the highest quartile, with triglycerides of, say, 190 and HDL of 37, even an ideal cholesterol count of 180 leaves you at great risk. But if your triglyceride level is no higher than your HDL, then a total cholesterol of even 300 may mean very little heart risk.

It's pretty obvious, then, that your ratio of triglycerides to HDL cholesterol is critically important to your future heart health. Ideally, you want a ratio approaching 1:1, with your triglycerides lower than your HDL. If your ratio is 2:1, with your triglycerides higher than your HDL, you're on the borderline of normal. Anything higher than 2:1 begins to be serious if you're over the 100-mg/dL mark for triglycerides. You're asking for heart trouble, trouble that simple dietary changes could help you avoid completely.

And what is the change? In many of my patients, a low-carbohydrate diet, combined with such vitanutrients as omega-3 fatty acids and vitamin C, has made their high triglycerides plummet by 60 or even 80 percent in just a few weeks. The dietary change didn't originate with me. It's been well-known, even if the conclusion is largely ignored, since the publication of a paper on the subject by P. K. Reissell's group at Harvard in 1966. The study demonstrated dramatic and consistent corrections of severely elevated triglyceride levels with a diet strikingly similar to the induction phase—very low-carbohydrate—of the Atkins diet.[7]

The reason has to do with the glycemic index, a standard scale used to measure the ability of carbohydrate-containing foods to elevate blood sugar and insulin levels. (More about insulin in the next chapter.) On the glycemic index, a slice of white bread is the standard food; it's given the scale number of 100. The lower the number, the lower the glycemic index of the food. Beans and lentils, for instance, are much lower on the scale than bread, sweets, and potatoes, but meat, eggs, fish, and fowl are virtually zero.

Foods high on the glycemic index—primarily refined or simple carbohydrates taken without protein or fat to buffer their response—are known to cause an excessive outpouring of insulin, which in turn raises the triglyceride level. A very significant 1999 study confirmed this fact.[8]

I've confirmed it, too: Long-term Atkins dieters, who eat foods low on the glycemic index, consistently develop higher HDL levels and lower TG levels.

(Note that timing is important when you go for a triglycerides blood test. Unlike cholesterol, which isn't really affected by eating, your triglyceride level can jump sharply after you eat. Schedule your test for first thing in the morning, and don't eat anything or drink anything other than plain water for ten to twelve hours before.)

Why are triglyceride elevations so much more likely to lead to heart disease when they are combined with low levels of HDL than when they are not? I can't give you an absolute answer. Theorists postulate that whatever causes triglyceride elevation will, if profound enough, interfere with the synthesis of HDL cholesterol.

Whatever the final answer, my evidence of the truth of the matter lies in the more than 30,000 before-and-after lipid profiles the Atkins Center has done on patients pre- and post-carbohydrate restriction. Those with elevated triglycerides get a 60 to 80 percent drop in their triglycerides, combined with a 15 to 30 percent increase in their HDL. My data are only retrospective and thus are of less scientific value than a controlled, double-blind study would be. Should the day come when someone replicates these findings (I have no doubt that any study will get the same results), this is what they will prove: *Both elevated triglycerides and low levels of HDL come from the overconsumption of refined carbohydrates and are correctable by the restriction of carbohydrates.*

LIPOPROTEIN(a)

Lipoprotein(a) is as good a leading predictor of heart disease as high triglycerides. This is a blood fat to take very seriously. Lp(a) is actually a type of LDL cholesterol that's very sticky. The molecules of Lp(a) attach to the LDL particles in your blood and give you a double whammy. Because they're so sticky, Lp(a) particles can cause blockages and clots in your arteries. Even worse, they can keep plasminogen, your body's natural clot-dissolving enzyme, from working properly. That means the clot could further damage your artery or even cause a heart attack.

A reading of 20 mg/dL is a normal Lp(a) level. Anything between 20 and 30 mg/dL is borderline, and anything above 30 mg/dL is elevated.

If your Lp(a) is on the high side, it could be genetic predisposition. But it's more likely that your elevated level is caused by what you eat. We know that one of the major causes of high lipoprotein(a) levels is eating large amounts of hydrogenated and partially hydrogenated fats—the dreaded trans fats I'll discuss at length in Chapter 14. We also know that a good way to lower your Lp(a) level is to eat more saturated fats. If you throw out margarine and switch to butter, then you're making a good start on lowering your Lp(a) level.

You might be wondering why your body naturally makes something as potentially harmful as Lp(a). What good does it do? That's a question the great chemist and two-time Nobel laureate Linus Pauling asked himself. His answer is interesting. Pauling remembered that humans and other primates—along with fruit-eating bats and guinea pigs—are among the very few animals that can't make their own vitamin C. Instead, they must obtain it from the foods they eat. And these same animals are also the only ones to have lipoprotein(a) in their blood. Pauling noted that, in normal amounts, Lp(a) works to keep your blood vessels strong, protects your arteries from damage, and helps repair any damage that does occur—exactly the same thing that vitamin C does, among many other crucial roles in your body. For this reason, Pauling, along with his colleague Dr. Mathias Rath, theorized that Lp(a) is a sort of fallback mechanism for times when we have a shortage of vitamin C.

To prove their theory, Pauling and Rath first caused atherosclerosis in guinea pigs and then kept them from getting any vitamin C. In the absence of vitamin C, the plaque accumulated Lp(a). When the guinea pigs were given plenty of vitamin C, however, they didn't develop any plaque in their damaged arteries.[9]

What the Pauling-Rath theory suggests is that high levels of vitamin C—perhaps as high as several grams a day—keep lipoprotein(a) in check. Combined with a diet that's low in trans fats and high in saturated fats, and along with some other vitanutrients such as niacin and N-acetyl-cysteine, you could lower your Lp(a) level naturally.

HOMOCYSTEINE: THE HIDDEN HEART HARMER

If the lipid profile contains the most important and prevalent heart risk, there's another important risk to be discussed. It's perhaps the most unnecessary risk: elevated levels of an abnormal protein called homocysteine.

A normal by-product of metabolizing the amino acid methionine, homocysteine is usually cleared rapidly from your blood before it can damage your arteries. In some people, though, homocysteine levels become dangerously elevated. Most studies of the causes of heart disease seem to agree that about 10 percent of coronary deaths and a somewhat greater proportion of stroke deaths can be directly attributed to abnormally high levels of homocysteine. This translates into more than 100,000 deaths in the United States every year, many of them in people who had perfectly fine blood lipid levels and no other risk factors for heart disease.

More to the point, homocysteine may be one of the direct causes of aging itself. Australian researcher Michael Fenech, using the technique of measuring micronuclei in human lymphocytes as an indication of damage to chromosomes (a well-accepted cause of aging), found that higher homocysteine levels resulted in increased chromosomal damage.[10]

Homocysteine doesn't come from eating eggs or saturated fat; in fact, it doesn't come from what you eat at all. It results from what you *don't* eat. Simply put, elevated homocysteine is a vitamin deficiency. It comes from suboptimal blood levels of the B complex vitamins, especially folic acid, B_6, and/or B_{12}. You need these vitamins to make the enzymes that remove homocysteine from your body. When well-fed Americans still end up short on these crucial B vitamins, and when their doctors neglect to test for their homocysteine levels, it is the outrageous consequence of policy-makers' refusal to accept scientifically demonstrated information.

For decades, the U.S. government's Food and Drug Administration has placed a stringent limitation on the amount of folic acid, or folate, that could be legally permitted in a vitamin capsule. Even though numerous scientific studies have shown that folic acid is North America's number-one vitamin deficiency, is the single most important nutrient involved in homocysteine control, and is responsible for preventing serious birth defects, the FDA won't lift the scientifically insupportable restrictions. To this day folic acid is the only vitamin that carries any dosage limitation.

Here's the irony: Every single one of the deaths attributed to homocysteine elevations could have been easily prevented had those people taken folic acid supplements in sufficient amounts. Why didn't they? An explanation is very much in order.

The homocysteine risk was first called to the public's attention by Dr. Kilmer McCully in the late 1960s. He pointed out not only that this compound was causing fatal heart attacks from damaged blood vessels, but also that it could always be normalized by taking adequate amounts of folic acid plus B_6 and B_{12}.

Consider the impact of McCully's well-conducted research. Here was a major cause of heart deaths that would not sell corn oil, cereal, margarine, or drugs; it would sell vitamins.

So the countercurrent swung into action. McCully was let go from his position as pathologist, he was denied tenure, and he saw his work branded as insignificant. It took fifteen years, during which time an estimated 1.5 million Americans died of homocysteine-related vascular disease, before numerous reports confirmed McCully's work and found that levels of homocysteine previously considered normal were capable of tripling the incidence of heart disease. What we still don't know is exactly how homocysteine damages your arteries, but damage them it most certainly does.

Let's look at two recent studies that show just how important it is to keep your homocysteine level low. In 1997, a large European trial found that among men and women younger than sixty, the overall risk of coronary and other vascular disease was 2.2 times higher in those with plasma homocysteine levels in the top fifth of the normal range than in those in the bottom four-fifths. The risk was independent of other factors, but it was notably higher in smokers and people with high blood pressure.[11]

Even mildly elevated homocysteine levels increase your chances of death from any cause, not just heart disease. In a long-term study of nearly 2,000 residents of western Jerusalem, the risk of death was twice as high among subjects with the highest levels of homocysteine as among those with the lowest levels. Subjects with mildly to moderately elevated homocysteine levels had a 30 to 50 percent higher risk of death than those with lowest levels.[12]

Not all our failures to avail ourselves of the scientific discoveries that can make our lives easier—and longer— can be attributed so clearly. But there are real villains in the homocysteine story. Taking a properly dosed multiple vitamin with enough folic acid could virtually eliminate anyone's homocysteine-based problem. Yet the American Heart Association and an entire roster of similar groups have never wavered from their position that vitamins should come from the food we eat and should not be taken as supplements. To prove my point, here's the official American Heart Association recommendation on homocysteine, quoted verbatim: "Although evidence for the benefit of lowering homocysteine levels is lacking, patients at high risk should be strongly advised to follow an overall diet that ensures adequate intake of folic acid and vitamins B_6 and B_{12}."[13] Meanwhile, surveys in both the United States and Canada have fingered folic acid as the number-one vitamin deficiency of all.

Another villain in the story has a fifty-year history of fighting folic acid by limiting its legal dosage to 0.8 mg, a quantity that is often not adequate to correct homocysteine elevations. I'm speaking, of course, of the FDA.

Thanks to this agency, an individual savvy enough to take a daily multivitamin is unlikely to get enough folic acid to render homocysteine innocuous, because of those FDA regulations that forbid putting in enough to make a difference. The specious rationale is that taking large doses of folic acid could mask a deficiency of vitamin B_{12}. The problem, if it is one, could easily be circumvented by simply testing for vitamin B_{12} before starting the folic acid. Hundreds of daily vitamin-takers have come to me with elevated homocysteine levels, only to have them normalized when prescription-strength folic acid was given.

It is my hope that the evidence proving the opposite of the FDA antifolate position will get out: Everyone should be taking folic acid in amounts large enough to prevent heart disease.

Let's summarize what I've discussed so far and see what it tells us about heart disease and nutrition.

We know that whatever is causing today's heart disease epidemic was not there eighty or more years ago. Rather, heart attacks are a modern phenomenon that occur in Western or Westernized cultures.

We know Cleave's Rule of Twenty Years and its warning that whenever refined carbohydrates become a major addition to a culture, coronary heart disease and diabetes begin to appear in two decades.

We know that the ratio of blood lipid levels most likely to eventuate in a heart attack is the combination of high triglycerides and low HDL cholesterol.

And we know that a couple of other key heart-disease predictors in the blood—high Lp(a) and high homocysteine—can be turned around with simple vitamin intake.

What do all these important facts have in common? What do they tell you about reversing heart disease?

I'll take my time explaining my answer in the following chapters, but all these facts point to one pretty simple idea: There is a direct correlation between nutrition and the disease that prematurely ages more of us than anything else. The facts also point to one fairly simple solution: If we rethink nutrition—both what we eat and the vitanutrients that can supplement what we eat—we may be able to eradicate the disease and dramatically turn back the clock.

To do that, we need first to understand the role of a real culprit in the aging process—insulin. If you thought insulin was just something diabetics had to have, read on.

5

WHY WE AGE: THE INSULIN CONNECTION

There are some fifteen million diabetics in the United States today. Perhaps four times that number of people, however, are prediabetic; that is, their bodies aren't responding to insulin or not using it properly or they are making too much of it, or not enough. What does this have to do with aging and with learning how to defy the effects of aging? A great deal, as it turns out.

Remember Cleave's research and his finding that the consumption of refined carbohydrates in a typical Westernized diet invariably led to both heart disease and diabetes, as well as to an array of other degenerative diseases? It's time now to explore that further and to learn why heart disease and diabetes are so inextricably linked; why what ultimately links them is diet, specifically, a diet high in carbohydrates; and why the refining of carbohydrates is in reality the greatest *unacknowledged* cause of death in world history.

We'll look first at the disease diabetes itself and how it progresses. Then we'll explore the how and why of the insulin connection: the effects of insulin levels on the body's own functioning, hypertension, and the production of essential hormones. Keep in mind as you go through this discussion that it is the carbohydrate content of our typical Western diet that is the first cause of these effects. By the end of the chapter, you'll have a good idea of how much bad health and premature aging we can avoid or prevent if we only reduce that carbohydrate intake.

HEART DISEASE AND DIABETES: THE LINK

Type II diabetes, also known as adult-onset or noninsulin-dependent diabetes, affects 95 percent of the fifteen million diabetics in America. The additional 60 million Americans who are very likely prediabetic are afflicted, whether they know it or not, with some form of insulin disorder. These disorders progress in stages from insulin resistance to a diagnosis of full-blown diabetes. Each stage has its own particular problems, and each opens a door—a little wider with every progression—to the range of degenerative diseases we associate with aging. So a discussion of the stages of this disease, technical though it may be, will help you understand the inexorable connections among carbohydrates, disease, and aging.

Stage 1: Insulin Resistance

Insulin is a hormone made in the pancreas whose major role is to convert excess sugar, or glucose, into a stored form of energy called glycogen. Glycogen is an essential body fuel, but excess glycogen can be converted into stored fat in the form of triglycerides. In stage 1 diabetes, the cells in the pancreas that produce insulin are destroyed. The result is a total failure to produce insulin, and the essential job of converting glucose to glycogen goes undone. This is called insulin resistance, and while it is a condition unto itself, it usually leads to stage 2 of the disease. In fact, because insulin resistance is hard to diagnose in normal medical practice—it requires us to measure glucose simultaneously from an artery and vein of the same leg—we typically diagnose it by inference after noting weight gain or a finding of stage 2.

Stage 2: Hyperinsulinism

In stage 2, the problem is not insulin resistance but excessive insulin—hyperinsulism. And thereby hangs a tale.

The big breakthrough in understanding diabetes was the technology for measuring serum insulin levels. Much to everyone's surprise, it was quickly discovered that type II diabetics were the polar opposite of type I insulin-dependent diabetics. Type IIs put out *too much* insulin, often more than persons with insulin-secreting tumors; type I diabetics, because they have a damaged pancreas, don't put out any insulin.

Here we see the twentieth century's crosscurrents at work again. The scientific community clearly demonstrated that the two illnesses sharing the name "diabetes" were completely different illnesses, type I coming from insulin *lack* and type II deriving from insulin *resistance*. The truth-suppressing crosscurrent, in this instance from the American Diabetes Association, erroneously insists that the two are variants of the same disease, and that type II patients should be treated with insulin or insulin-releasing drugs.

Shortly after the discovery that insulin levels could be measured, it was established that stage 2 hyperinsulinism could itself lead to heart disease and other illnesses. Dr. Gerald Reaven of Stanford University, a prominent researcher in this field, summarized the impact of hyperinsulinism as a collection of features he dubbed Syndrome X: abdominal obesity (our single most prevalent abnormality, as I'm sure you've noticed), hypertension, a variety of blood sugar abnormalities, and two heart risk factors, high triglycerides and low HDL cholesterol.

Now, if you are the kind of reader who likes to form conclusions *while* you are reading, I'll wager you have been startled by what I just wrote. Feel free to exclaim what's going through your mind: "The link between diabetes and heart disease begins with the second stage of diabetes. Diabetes causes heart disease before it is recognized as diabetes!" Congratulations—you've caught on.

Stage 3: Blood Sugar Abnormalities

Diagnosing the very common blood sugar abnormalities of stage 3 requires a glucose tolerance test, or GTT, a test of such importance that I have ordered it for more than 40,000 Atkins Center patients. The patient takes glucose orally, and the GTT shows when the insulin disorder begins to affect the blood sugar's response to the glucose. Sometimes, the abnormality appears at the beginning of the test, as the blood glucose rises to a point higher than that of a normal person, where "normal" is generally considered to be 160 mg/dL. More often, the abnormality appears on the downslope, when, presumably affected by the increased quantity or effectiveness of the insulin hyperactivity, the glucose level drops at a rate exceeding 50 points in a single hour, or 100 points in all.

Interpreting the GTT can be a fairly subjective process, but most of the time it's perfectly obvious when the criteria of abnormality are exceeded in a major way. I always administer the GTT in conjunction with a symptom questionnaire, because the symptoms of blood sugar instability noticed by the patient are every bit as important in establishing a diagnosis as is the GTT.

Among these symptoms are hour-by-hour changes in

energy level, mood, brain function, and irritability—often brought on by being somewhat hungry, and just as often relieved by food or caffeine. Carbohydrate cravings, voracious hunger, and excessive tiredness are also commonly noted.

If your dietary habits include lots of refined carbohydrates, fruit juices, caffeine, sweets, or alcohol, the suspicion that you may be in the third stage—the last prediabetic stage—may serve you just as well as the certainty of a GTT. If the suspicion leads you to change your errant ways, it will achieve the desired end of preventing you from progressing to the fourth stage of prediabetes.

Remember that stage 3 of prediabetes is quite common. I see bona fide abnormalities in GTTs in my patients about four times more often than I see diabetes. That would suggest that one third of the American population has this problem. Once you know you have the problem and make the necessary dietary changes and take the appropriate vitanutrients, you are very unlikely to progress to stage 4.

Stage 4: Recognizable Type II Diabetes

There is rarely a noticeable difference between stage 3 and the typical stage 4 type II diabetes. No new symptoms develop, there is little if any change in the excessive body weight that plagues over 80 percent of these people, and there is almost never a worsening of heart symptoms. It's simply that now the blood sugars are generally elevated throughout the day. The insulin resistance and hyperinsulinism that defined stages 1 through 3 are still there.

That means that type II diabetes responds to the same low-carbohydrate diet and vitanutrients that bring the prediabetic stages under control. The countercurrent that denies these science-based facts? Your diabetologist is almost certain to recommend continuance of your high-carbohydrate food consumption; he or she is almost equally certain to prescribe drugs—usually those which increase your insulin levels and, according to a well-conducted 1970 study, increase your likelihood of a fatal heart attack by 150 percent.

Not all stage 4 diabetics continue to put out excessive insulin throughout their illness. They do, however, continue to have blood sugar elevations for the reason common to all five stages of type II: They are insulin-resistant. It is not until this late stage of diabetes that insulin output begins to be inadequate—and insulin failure leads to stage 5.

Stage 5: Diabetes, Type II, with Low Insulin
Diabetologists who confuse type I with type II diabetes are justified in their error only when stage 5 is reached. By this point in a type II diabetic's life, his or her insulin output has finally become subnormal.

At the Atkins Center, we routinely test our type II diabetics by drawing insulin levels before and after a high-carbohydrate test breakfast. If there is any elevation of insulin after the meal, it can come only from a functioning pancreas. In our diabetic patients, only 10 percent put out insulin levels so inadequate they can't be managed without an insulin supplement.

The countercurrent? Some 44 percent of type II diabetics who consult diabetes specialists are prescribed insulin. The Atkins Center experience has shown that the majority of them are given insulin unnecessarily.

THE INSULIN/AGING CONNECTION

I told you the discussion would be technical. I think it's helpful, however, in understanding why avoiding diabetes-related illness is likely to be the most important key to avoiding aging.

Simply put, here's why: We've just seen that a type II diabetic goes through three prediabetic stages prior to becoming a diabetic. All of these prediabetic stages are associated with an excessive insulin outpouring when carbohydrates are consumed. That is, they are all stages of hyperinsulinism, and one of the effects of hyperinsulinism is the production of high triglycerides and low HDL cholesterol. This deadly combination, as we know from the previous chapter, is the most predictive risk factor for atherosclerosis, and atherosclerosis is the great aging disease of our time and place. QED: Hyperinsulinism, or prediabetes, and refined carbohydrates have an awfully strong connection with shortening human life spans.

I cannot claim to be the first to espouse the theory. That honor belongs to a world-famous Russian scientist, Dr. Vladimir Dilman, of St. Petersburg. In a series of books and scientific papers, Professor Dilman presented a comprehensive theory that the symptoms of aging are caused mainly by hyperinsulinism. So convinced was he of insulin's role in aging that the major pharmaceutical he recommended for antiaging purposes was the only drug then available—metformin, an oral medication that works by overcoming insulin resistance. Professor Dilman's successful research outcomes with this drug became the basis of his conclusions about the need to overcome insulin resistance and its inseparable companion, hyperinsulinism.

Professor Dilman was a pioneer, and his theories, arrived at thirty to forty years ago, form the intellectual scaffolding for the vast amount of scientific research that has come since then. I met him in New York City toward the end of his career, which he had decided to close. When he arrived, he called me to introduce himself. He told me that as far as he was concerned, I was the only American doctor who seemed to be on the right track, and he said he would like to work with me in doing further research on longevity. I was more than flattered, but I had to inform the professor that the Atkins Center is not set up as a research facility—our function is strictly to help our patients get and stay well. We stayed in touch nonetheless until his untimely death in the 1970s. He greatly influenced my thinking about how to defy age, and much of what he taught me is still relevant in the fight against aging today.

The research on insulin and aging continues, of course. As I write this book, researchers at Harvard University are conducting the ongoing New England Centenarian Study, which has already produced some very interesting insulin-related results. One statistic from the study helps prove Dilman's point and mine. Of the 169 participants in the study—all of them people who have reached the age of at least 100 in fairly good health— only 6 have diabetes. That works out to only 3 percent of the total participants.[1] These people are living examples of how important it is to maintain good blood sugar control if we're going to defy aging.

Let's look at why.

HOW SWEET GOES SOUR

We'll begin with glucose, the sugar substance your body uses as the main fuel for its operations. Where does the fuel come from? Mostly from carbohydrates in the food you eat. Your body converts these carbohydrates into sugars, and the glucose enters your bloodstream. That increase in your blood sugar level alerts the portion of your pancreas known as the islets of Langerhans to start pouring out insulin.

The insulin's job is to control the distribution of all that sugar. It carries some of it into your cells, where it is then taken up by the mitochondria, tiny structures within the cells that act as little power plants to burn the glucose for fueling the body's activity. Some of the sugar that's not needed immediately is converted to glycogen, a starch that's stored in your muscles and liver and that serves as your body's spare gas tank, able to provide quick energy when it's needed. The glycogen storage areas fill up pretty quickly, though. We have only a two-day glycogen supply. The sugar that's left in your blood at that point gets converted by insulin into the tiny fat particles we know as triglycerides, which are what your body fat is made from and which, as we know, are about as predictive a risk factor for heart disease as you can find.

So far, so good. Your body uses insulin to keep your blood sugar within a fairly narrow range, generally between 65 and 100 mg per 100 cc of blood. That's the level your body works best at, and it's the level that millions of years of evolution have designed your body to maintain.

But evolution is a slow process. For while your body is perfectly adapted to eat the foods that were the mainstay of existence for the vast length of human history—fats and proteins from animal foods and unrefined carbohydrates from plant foods—it doesn't do as well with today's processed foods. Your body does fine with fats, which have virtually no effect on your blood sugar and insulin levels, and with proteins, which have very little effect. Similarly, unrefined carbohydrates from fruits, vegetables, and whole grains are relatively low in carbohydrates and release their sugar slowly into your blood.* The body does fine with them, too.

But our bodies were never meant to cope with the huge amounts of refined carbohydrates we eat today, mostly in the form of sugar, especially table sugar and high-fructose corn syrup, skim milk, fruit juice, dried fruit, and white flour in bread, baked goods, pasta, and the like, and other starchy foods like baked potatoes and white rice. This is a diet that plays havoc with our blood sugar and our insulin.

Eating the typical high-carbohydrate American diet forces the body constantly to produce large amounts of insulin to cope with all that glucose. If you eat that typical diet in the typically large portions that your countrymen consume, you're going to have a lot of leftover glucose in your blood, which your insulin will promptly convert to fat. Now the vicious cycle really sets in, because the fatter you get, the less responsive to insulin your cells become. While eating the carbohydrates triggers your body increasingly to release insulin, your cells

*How slowly varies, depending on the food. The effect of individual foods on your sugar and insulin levels is quantified by a system called the glycemic index. See page 360 for a list of the glycemic index values of a variety of foods.

increasingly don't want to let it in. This is called insulin resistance, and you'll recall that that's also the description of stage 1 in type II diabetes.

Once insulin resistance sets in, your body, in an effort to maintain its normal equilibrium, produces even more insulin to overcome the resistance. Because the insulin can't carry much glucose into your cells to be burned as fuel, the glucose remains in your blood instead. Insulin converts some of the excess sugar to fat. You get fatter, and you also feel tired all the time, partly because your cells aren't getting the fuel they need, and partly because the excess insulin drives your blood sugar below the optimal range. Your body can't convert all that excess sugar into fat fast enough to keep it from circulating in your blood. The result can be very damaging, and your heart, blood vessels, kidneys, eyes, and nerves are particularly vulnerable.

As you slide farther down the slippery slope of insulin resistance, you're constantly putting out insulin to no good effect. In fact, it's doing serious damage to your body. You've developed hyperinsulinism: Your insulin is always too high even as your body is resistant to its effects. That equates to the second stage of type II diabetes.

If you're not overweight, you're probably thinking, "Well, I'm safe. No blood sugar worries for me." I'm sorry to tell you that you're not safe at all. The mere fact of growing older means your cells are becoming at least somewhat resistant to glucose. About 25 percent of all apparently healthy, normal-weight adults are nonetheless affected by insulin resistance. Among people who smoke and/or have a sedentary lifestyle, the percentage is even higher. So such people are just as likely to move to the next step in the progression, stage 3 or impaired glucose tolerance. This abnormality is said to affect 11 percent of the healthy adult population, but the number is actually considerably more. In my experience, which includes reviewing more than 45,000 glucose tolerance tests, abnormal glucose responses outnumber diabetes by three to one. That places the number of adults with impaired glucose tolerance at closer to 30 percent of the population (10 percent of the adult population has diabetes). This implies that nearly half of all adults, by the time they reach the age of fifty, will demonstrate at least some instability in their blood sugar and at least some insulin resistance. Of course, if you're considerably overweight, your chances of having insulin resistance, hyperinsulinism, and eventual diabetes are approaching near certainty.

THE AGING EXPRESS LANE

Now do you see why I insisted on describing all the stages of diabetes? It comes down to this: Hyperinsulinism accelerates aging. Even small elevations in glucose and insulin levels affect your health as you age and are closely related to the chronic disorders of aging, including heart disease, cancer, and of course diabetes.[2]

That alone should be enough to convince you that blood sugar control must be at the core of any age-defying program. But given that more than half of all American adults are overweight, that nearly 20 million Americans have been diagnosed with diabetes, that diabetes now kills one American every three minutes, and that the disease is in the process of exploding to epidemic levels, with 300 million cases projected worldwide twenty-five years hence, let me bring home the dangers of hyperinsulinism even more fully.

As we saw in the description of the five stages of

diabetes, the middle three stages are all associated with excessively high levels of insulin, particularly when stimulated by the intake of carbohydrates. Because the insulin disorder precedes the diagnosable stage of diabetes by anywhere from two years to forty years (twenty years is the average) and because the insulin disorder does not always progress to diabetes, there are far more people with hyperinsulinism than with diabetes. If we accept the conservative estimate that hyperinsulinism is four times as common as diabetes, that means that the 300 million cases of diabetes projected worldwide for 2025 would translate into 1.2 *billion* cases of too much insulin.

It's not just an issue of normal versus abnormal. There are many gradations of glucose and insulin levels, and each gradation has its own danger level. For instance, if your fasting glucose is in the upper range of normal, you have a substantially higher risk of death from heart disease than someone at the lower end of normal. In fact, if you're a middle-aged man with a fasting blood glucose level between 85 and 109 mg/dL, your heart risk is 40 percent higher than average. You also have a greater chance of several other unfavorable cardiovascular risk factors, including high blood pressure and high LDL cholesterol and triglycerides.[3]

You can also go beyond simply being at the high end to having impaired glucose tolerance. This applies to people with a fasting blood glucose level that is higher than 110 mg/dL but is not yet at the diabetic level of above 125. Those people are at even greater risk for cardiovascular disease,[4] and I am sure that future studies will confirm that insulin gradations within the normal range are just as predictive of these problems as is glucose.

So just how do glucose intolerance and hyperinsulinism affect how we age?

HOW SUGAR MAKES US AGE

I've told you that elevated blood sugar levels are bad for you. I've told you that diabetics don't live as long as other people and that very few centenarians are diabetics—but I didn't tell you why. It's because of the adverse effect that blood sugar elevations have on our body's organs. The process whereby sugar does that is called glycosylation. Once you know how glycosylation can hurt you, you may never enjoy another dessert again. The process has been well researched, but it's not widely known among the general public, so let me take some time to explain it to you.

Sugar is sticky, as you discover every time you spill some and have to wipe it up. When there's extra sugar floating around in your bloodstream, its sticky glucose molecules attach themselves to proteins. It's that attaching process that is known as glycosylation or, sometimes, glycation. When glycosylation happens in places where it doesn't belong, it sets in motion a slow chain of chemical reactions that ends with the proteins binding together, or cross-linking, and forming a new chemical structure. The brilliant biochemist Anthony Cerami, who discovered the glycosylation process in living tissue, gave these new structures a very apt name: Advanced Glycosylation End-products, or AGEs.

Why are AGEs so dangerous? Here's an analogy that may make it clearer: What's happening to your tissues from exposure to excess glucose is exactly what happens to meat when you brown it. You're slowly cooking yourself from the inside. Glycosylation alters the very structure of proteins and keeps them from doing what they're supposed to do.

Collagen is one of the first proteins to be affected. Collagen is the tough but flexible connective tissue that holds your skeleton together, attaching your muscles to your bones and serving as the foundation of all your blood vessels, your skin, your lungs, and your cartilage. When collagen becomes glycosylated and AGEs form, the cross-linking destroys collagen's flexibility. This means that your blood vessels, lungs, and joints all stiffen; your skin sags; the proteins in the lens of your eye cloud over, resulting in cataracts.

Other proteins are also affected by AGEs. For example, glucose easily combines with the protein hemoglobin in your blood. In fact, that potential combination is the basis of a valuable blood test for diabetes, called glycosylated hemoglobin (GHb). GHb measures your blood sugar average over several consecutive months and can tell us how much AGEing you have done over that time span.

AGEs also affect the more than 50,000 different proteins your body makes to regulate how it functions. For example, your body produces antioxidant enzymes that protect you against free radicals. When glucose attaches to these enzymes, they become inactive; the AGEs destroy the mechanism that produces these enzymes. As we'll see in more detail in the following chapter, even slight elevations in your blood sugar are enough to produce excess free radicals—more than your body can cope with. Indeed, the overabundance of free radicals is one of the primary reasons for the accelerated aging often seen in diabetics. And because vitamin C is carried into your cells along with insulin, one consequence of even slight insulin resistance is that you'll have less of this powerful antioxidant in your cells.

Other proteins are part of complex chemical cascades that send messages around your body, turning genes on and off, repairing damage, and controlling the growth and replication of cells. When these controlling proteins are damaged by AGEs, the chemical messages become garbled or fail to get through at all. When that happens, the proper functioning of the cell is disrupted, and that in turn causes further disruption down the message line. If the disruption causes a gene to switch on or off inappropriately, or if it tells a cell to replicate when it shouldn't, the result can set in motion the process that leads to cancer and other problems.

It's possible that AGEs can even bind directly to the DNA in a cell's nucleus. Although the process would happen very slowly, over the long run it would cause serious damage in cells that don't reproduce, such as those in your heart and brain.

Sticky AGEs also tend to form clumps of cross-linked proteins that are very similar to the tangles and plaques found in the brains of Alzheimer's patients. Indeed, AGEs have been found in these plaques at about three times the level in normal brains, suggesting that they are responsible, at least in part, for the progression of this dreadful disease.[5]

When glucose attaches to the tiny protein molecules known as peptides, the resulting AGEs end up circulating in your blood. This can have an adverse effect on your blood lipids, because the AGE-modified peptides may then attach to molecules of LDL cholesterol. When that happens, as recent research suggests, the body fails to recognize this new substance as LDL. As a result, the LDL stays in circulation instead of being removed from your blood as part of the normal clearance process. This explains in part why diabetics have such dangerously high levels of LDL cholesterol—all the extra sugar in their blood leads to high levels of circulating AGEs.[6]

Your body does have some natural defenses against AGEs. At least one type of scavenger cell in your immune system engulfs and destroys AGEs, but the process doesn't seem to be very efficient, and it slows down even more with age. Your antioxidant enzymes may also play a part in keeping AGEs to a minimum.

Interestingly, AGEs may explain the beneficial effect on the heart of having a daily cocktail or glass of wine. The alcohol seems to block the formation of some AGEs at an intermediate stage in the process, keeping them from building up inside your arteries and damaging your LDL cholesterol.[7]

HYPERTENSION

Here's another way that insulin resistance and glucose intolerance conspire to age you: They raise your blood pressure. It's well-known, of course, that sharply higher blood pressure is one of the most serious consequences of diabetes and puts the diabetic at far greater risk of heart disease, stroke, and kidney disease. But you don't have to be diabetic to get blood pressure elevations; the insulin disorders that appear long before diabetes does will do the trick.[8] In fact, Stanford's Dr. Reaven suggests that 60 percent of hypertension cases can be attributed to hyperinsulinism.

A conventional doctor will probably tell you that your blood pressure is going up simply because you're getting older. And in fact, elevated blood pressure among older adults is so common that it's called age-related hypertension. When it happens to you, you've reached the stage in life that the drug companies love. Now they can look forward to having you as a lifelong customer of medications that lower blood pressure, including diuretics and beta-blockers. My prescription, however, when it comes to these drugs, is to just say no. I've treated more than 10,000 patients who were taking blood pressure medications, and I've seen nutritional changes help them get off their medications permanently. Instead, we consistently bring high blood pressure right back down to normal by reducing the carbohydrates in the patient's diet—thus returning blood glucose and insulin to better levels—and by adding such vitanutrients as taurine, magnesium, potassium, coenzyme Q_{10}, hawthorn, and garlic. Of course, if you're overweight, shedding those excess pounds will also help return your blood pressure to normal.

DHEA DISTURBANCES

Dehydroepiandrosterone (DHEA) is a critically important hormone for defying the aging process, as I'll discuss in greater detail in Chapter 12. The point that belongs in this chapter, however, is that a rising insulin level causes your DHEA to drop.

Here too, the effects are seen long before diabetes develops. If you're at the high end of normal DHEA levels, lowering your insulin level will still increase your DHEA.[9] If your DHEA levels are high, you're much less likely to develop diabetes to begin with. That's because DHEA improves insulin resistance, even in people who already have diabetes.[10] Interestingly, chromium picolinate, a supplement we often use at the Atkins Center to improve the insulin resistance of diabetic patients, also seems to increase your production of DHEA by lowering your blood levels of insulin.[11]

But one of the best ways by far to keep your DHEA level from dipping into the inadequate range is to avoid even a "high normal" insulin level, because that, more than anything else, will suppress your natural DHEA production.

DEALING WITH THE INSULIN/BLOOD SUGAR DILEMMA

Clearly, insulin resistance can open the door to all the degenerative diseases we think of as common to aging: diabetes, atherosclerosis, obesity, hypertension, impaired immunity, osteoporosis, even cancer. But the truth is that these diseases are not inevitable consequences of aging.

Instead, in almost all cases, they are the accumulated consequences of high blood sugar and high insulin. That makes them far from inevitable—indeed, they can all be prevented and even reversed. How? For most sufferers of the disease as well as most medical practitioners, the question presents a dilemma. Here's the problem.

Obviously, too much insulin in the blood can have harmful effects. So can too much sugar in the blood. Yet it is insulin that brings blood sugar back to normal. Ideally, that insulin comes from the individual's own body, but in the case of diabetics, it comes from the insulin a doctor prescribes.

Patients are asked to choose which is the better strategy: bring the sugar down or keep the insulin dose down. I can tell you what most doctors do: They worry about the sugar and give the insulin. Some 44 percent of type II diabetics are given insulin. An even greater number are prescribed drugs that increase their insulin levels, even though most of them have excessively high insulin to begin with.

I don't mean to minimize the dilemma, for dilemma it is: Both insulin *and* glucose threaten the health of a diabetic. But I am suggesting that there's a third way to deal with the problem, an alternative that keeps us off both horns of the dilemma.

This alternative, although not obvious to many doctors, is almost laughably easy: Just keep both your blood sugar and insulin levels at the lower end of normal through a diet that is low in carbohydrates and high in antioxidants and vitanutrients.

Later in this book, you will learn exactly how this can be done. For now, we need to look at another important accelerator of the aging process: free radicals.

6

WHY WE AGE: FREE RADICALS

The words may conjure up a mental picture of long-haired student activists gathered at a demonstration, but free radicals are a lot more sinister than a bunch of kids rallying for a cause. In fact, the damage that free radicals can cause to the body is profound; as the damage accumulates, it becomes downright dangerous. There are many issues on which my colleagues in antiaging medicine and I disagree, but on free radicals we are pretty much unanimous: Damage from free radicals is at the core of the aging process.

It happens simply, although in a variety of ways and with a number of complex permutations: Free radicals attack and damage cells. The kind of damage they do, and the consequences of the damage, depends on the kind of cell attacked and its function in your body. If free radicals attack the fatty acids of a cell, the result could be "stickier" cholesterol. If the cell that is damaged is part of your genetic code, the result could be a botched cell replication process—and eventually, cancer.

That's why avoiding, minimizing, and counteracting the damaging effects of free radicals must be the fundamental principle of any age-defying program. Everything and anything you do to reduce the damage from free radicals will give you that much better chance of living your full life span with a minimum of disability.

The free radical theory of aging is so central to my age-defying diet that I'm using this whole chapter to explain it. I'll tell you what free radicals are and what they do, what causes them to attack and damage cells, and how we can fight back, countering their attack and controlling their deleterious effects on our body.

But first, some background on the theory itself.

THE FREE RADICAL THEORY OF AGING

I fully expect that the free radical theory of aging will be to life expectancy what the germ theory was to infectious disease. The germ theory, of course, is credited to the great French researcher Louis Pasteur, who claimed back in the 1870s that microscopically small organisms called germs were the cause of such illnesses as tuberculosis, cholera, smallpox, and the other infectious diseases that were the scourge of Pasteur's time. Of course, even for Pasteur, despite the mass of clear and convincing evidence he brought forth, it was years before the medical profession fully accepted his ideas. Once it did, the ideas kicked off a revolution in medicine and public health that changed the lives of people all over the world.

I believe we're on the threshold of another revolution in medicine today, one with an equally significant and wide-ranging impact. This revolution is also led by a great researcher, Dr. Denham Harman. Harman first proposed his Free Radical Theory of Aging[1] in 1954, but as with Pasteur's germ theory, it was ignored by most of the scientific establishment for some twenty years. The theory states that free radical reactions, which are a normal and unavoidable feature of metabolism, cause the slow deterioration of the body over time. The damage they do to cells destroys the body's ability to function, bit by bit. In short, the damage causes us to age.

Free radicals are especially likely to damage the mitochondria, the tiny energy-producing structures within our cells. The more damage to the mitochondria, the faster we age—and the more likely we are to develop an age-related disease such as high blood pressure or cancer.[2]

It sounds simple. Yet, just as the germ theory eventually led to the elimination of infectious disease as a leading cause of death, Harman's free radical theory, once it is finally accepted by the medical profession, could eventually lead to the slowing or elimination of age-related illnesses. And that in turn may well lead to huge increases in life span. Living in good health to the age of one hundred and beyond will become not just possible but common. For that, we'll owe Denham Harman the same universal acclamation we give to Louis Pasteur. Both will have succeeded in affecting our health and extending our lives for the better.

UNDERSTANDING FREE RADICALS

Remember high school chemistry? That's probably where you learned that an atom consists of a nucleus around which pairs of negatively charged electrons orbit. If one of the electrons in a pair is stripped away, the atom (or the molecule of which the atom is part) becomes unstable. It becomes highly reactive as it seeks to restore its energy balance by grabbing on to another electron—any electron, from anywhere. A highly reactive, out-of-balance atom or molecule with one or more unpaired electrons is known as a free radical.

Almost all living things, including plants, need oxygen to live. Every single cell in your body uses oxygen to create energy. How? Tiny structures in your cells— the mitochondria—use the oxygen to create adenosine triphosphate (ATP), the chemical substance that powers your cells. Without oxygen, the cell cannot create energy and simply dies.

The energy that's produced by the mitochondria keeps your body running, but along the way, the complex process of producing the energy uses free radicals. Most of the free radicals are contained within the reaction, but quite a few escape as a kind of "waste product." Think of the way your car engine burns gasoline and oxygen in the pistons to produce the energy that drives the automobile. That same process also produces such waste products as water vapor and carbon monoxide. When your body burns oxygen to create energy, the waste products are water and oxygen-based free radicals, also known as reactive oxygen species.

When the free radicals escape, they scurry around in your cell looking for another electron. A free radical might grab the electron from the cell membrane or perhaps from the DNA contained in the nucleus. Given that your body has about 60 trillion cells in it, you would think that the loss of a single electron wouldn't matter much; after all, how much damage could it do?

The damage accumulates. Every moment of every day, every one of the 60 trillion cells in your body is producing millions of free radicals. And when a free radical grabs an electron from a nearby molecule, it's only the start of a long cascade of damage. Yes, the molecule that lost the electron is damaged, but in addition, another free radical has been created. Each of those damages more healthy molecules. To go back to the car analogy, a free radical is like the first skid in what eventually becomes a pileup of smashed vehicles. In your body, what's left are a lot of damaged cells. The cumulative damage over years causes the diseases of aging.

Some free radical types are particularly dangerous. The superoxide free radical is created when oxygen is metabolized into ATP and water in your mitochondria. Even after the superoxide radical grabs an electron, it's still dangerous. In its reduced form, the superoxide radical goes on to react with hydrogen atoms and form hydrogen peroxide. Technically, hydrogen peroxide isn't a free radical, but it can trigger the formation of lots more free radicals. If those free radicals then react with iron or copper in your body, they produce an extremely reactive and very dangerous free radical called hydroxyl. Anthony Diplock, a major researcher into free radicals, says that "the hydroxyl radical can pluck an electron from almost any organic molecule in its vicinity, which will initiate further radical and nonradical processes that may lie at the heart of the etiogenesis [causation] of biochemical changes that will lead to disease."[3]

FREE RADICAL DAMAGE

When free radicals attack, they can damage any part of a cell. If the free radical attacks the fatty acids of the cell membrane, the cell can rupture. If the free radicals attack tiny enzyme storage structures in your cells called lysosomes, the lysosomes are released into the cell and destroy it, as well as nearby cells.

That's bad enough, but even worse is the process known as lipid peroxidation. As free radicals attack the fatty tissues throughout your body, they "hit" the tiny cholesterol droplets that float in your blood. When what they hit is the bad low-density cholesterol (LDL), it is oxidized. The result is that the cholesterol turns much stickier, so sticky that it then attaches to rough spots on the walls of your arteries. When that happens, plaque begins to form, and you're on the way to clogged arteries and a heart attack or stroke.

The DNA found in the nuclei of all your cells contains your genetic code. If it is attacked by free radicals, the code controlling the cell's replication can be damaged. Alternatively, the free radical might fuse the DNA with other proteins in the cell. Cross-linking, as this is called, prevents the cell from replicating altogether. In either case, whether the cell's replication is damaged or halted, the result could be cancer.

Most serious of all is free radical damage to your mitochondria. These amazing little structures are the powerhouses of our cells; they run a cell's machinery and are responsible for cell respiration, the extremely complex process of combining glucose, fats, and proteins with oxygen to release ATP and water. Some 90 percent of the oxygen you breathe ends up being processed in the mitochondria. Cell respiration takes place on the mitochondria's folded inner membrane, which is surrounded by a smooth outer membrane. Both membranes are very high in polyunsaturated fatty acids. As the respiratory routine proceeds apace on the inner membrane, free radicals in abundance are created—just a normal sideshow of the normal chain of events that creates energy.

Mitochondria have their own separate DNA that codes for the production of the thirteen mitochondrial proteins you need for cellular respiration. The DNA in the nuclei of your cells is intricately coiled and carefully packaged. Mitochondrial DNA is far more vulnerable—it's an almost unprotected ring.

Some of the superoxide free radicals used in cell respiration escape in the process—and as we grow older, more and more get away. The first organic structures they encounter are the fatty membranes of the mitochondria and the mitochondrial DNA. That means the mitochondria themselves are the most likely part of the cell to be damaged. Lipid peroxidation of the membranes can slow down or even stop energy production. Damage to the mitochondrial DNA also damages the inner membrane, because the DNA codes for the production of the proteins that create it.

Here's how Dr. Harman himself describes what happens: "It is likely that the life span of an individual is primarily determined by the rate of mitochondria damage, inflicted at an increasing rate with age by free radicals arising in the mitochondria in the course of normal respiration; this is reflected in decreases in adenosine triphosphate (ATP) production and increases in superoxide radical formation."[4] Eventually, as your mitochondria become less efficient from accumulated free radicals, a vicious cycle begins. You produce more and more superoxide radicals and have less and less defense against them. Eventually, your body's various defense mechanisms are simply overwhelmed by the free radicals.

OTHER SOURCES OF FREE RADICALS

Cell respiration isn't the only source of free radicals. Interestingly, your immune system has harnessed the destructive power of free radicals to destroy invaders. Your white blood cells attack invading pathogens by engulfing them and then blasting them with superoxide and hydrogen peroxide. That's fine, but it also means that any illness or infection creates a lot of extra free radicals; the longer you're sick, the more free radicals you create and the more damage they can do.

Many prescription drugs produce huge amounts of free radicals as they break down in your body. In other cases, the free radicals are produced by your liver trying to metabolize the drugs, part of the normal detoxification process the liver routinely carries out to remove waste products from your body. Moreover, many prescription and nonprescription drugs seriously deplete your antioxidant levels, depriving you of your natural defenses.

The foods you eat have a major effect on your production of free radicals. A big culprit here is polyunsaturated fat, especially when it's in the form of partially hydrogenated vegetable oil—the deadly trans fat. I'll get to trans fat later, but here I'll just let you know that consuming trans fats is guaranteed to make you produce more free radicals.

Free radicals are also generated in your body when you're exposed to normal background radiation and ultraviolet light from sunshine. Millions of years of evolution have made your body able to squelch most—though not all—of these free radicals. What the body is not very good at is dealing with all the pollutants that accompany life in the twenty-first century, including pesticides, herbicides, ozone, smog, cigarette smoke, soot, and automobile exhaust. Exposure to all these pollutants creates free radicals as your body tries to expel them.

It's also important to remember that exercise produces a lot of free radicals. In fact, it's not uncommon for highly conditioned athletes—marathon runners, for example—to suffer frequent colds and infections. These people train so hard and produce so many free radicals that they actually damage their own immune systems.

FIGHTING BACK

If free radicals are such normal and natural occurrences in the body, how can we possibly resist or reduce the damage they do?

There are two basic approaches. One is to prevent the formation of excess free radicals in the first place; the other is to neutralize their effect once they have escaped.

So far, we know of only one sure way to lower the production of free radicals: caloric restriction. The idea is that if you eat a lot less, you burn less fuel and create fewer free radicals. The caloric restriction theory is talked and written about more than any other antiaging theory, and I'll be discussing it in detail in the next chapter. It's logical, and it works on lab rats, but as I'll explain shortly, caloric restriction has never been shown to be effective in humans. It also has a number of serious drawbacks—aside from leaving you hungry all the time.

A more reasonable approach for preventing free radical formation is to avoid situations that increase the production of excess free radicals. That includes such specifics as avoiding pollutants and exercising moderately. Most important, it means staying healthy; in that way, you avoid the double whammy generation of extra free radicals—both from illness and from the drugs that "cure" the illness.

BREAKING THE CHAINS: ANTIOXIDANTS TO THE RESCUE

The most practical way to prevent free radical damage is to neutralize excess free radicals rapidly and thereby break the chain reaction process as quickly as possible. By quenching free radicals as soon as they're formed, you minimize the damage they can do. This chain-breaking approach is the very core of my age-defying program.

To break the chains of free radical damage and liberate yourself to achieve your maximum life span, you must take a two-pronged approach: Consume a diet high in antioxidant foods and take supplements of antioxidant vitanutrients.

You've no doubt heard a great deal about antioxidants in recent years. What are they? For one thing, they're a good example of the natural genius of the body, which evolved antioxidants to protect itself against the harmful effects of free radicals. How? An antioxidant quenches a free radical by donating to it the electron it seeks. The antioxidant thus stops the free radical in its tracks and halts the cascade of further free radical formation.

One reason humans have much longer life spans than other animals may be that we have extremely efficient antioxidant mechanisms, all designed to put a quick end to the free radical chain reaction. Your first line of defense is the powerful antioxidant enzymes your body makes, including superoxide dismutase (SOD), glutathione, and catalase. They're so important that we need to take a closer look at them.

ANTIOXIDANT ENZYMES AND VITANUTRIENTS

Let's start with SOD (superoxide dismutase). This is the enzyme that neutralizes the superoxide free radical that's produced so abundantly in your mitochondria. SOD breaks the free radical chain reaction by deconstructing the superoxide radical into oxygen and hydrogen peroxide. That's the first step.

The next step is to break up the hydrogen peroxide, because it's a free radical too, although a much less damaging one than the superoxide radical. To break down the hydrogen peroxide, your body uses another enzyme called catalase that turns the hydrogen peroxide into plain water and oxygen. The catch here is that catalase works only in the watery parts of your body—inside your cells and outside your cells but not in the fatty cell membrane.

That's where the antioxidant enzyme glutathione comes in. It captures the free radicals attacking your cell membranes and also picks up any hydrogen peroxide your catalase misses. That's important, because hydrogen peroxide can break down into hydroxyl, the most dangerous free radical of all. Unfortunately, your body doesn't have an enzyme system for getting rid of hydroxyl. All it can do is to neutralize hydroxyl with the natural hormone melatonin. But as you'll learn in greater detail in Chapter 9, your production of melatonin drops as you age. We can and do raise the melatonin level with supplements, but a better method is to prevent hydroxyl radicals from forming.

We know from research that grows more definitive all the time that vitanutrients are essential for free radical protection. Such antioxidant nutrients as vitamin E, vitamin C, and beta-carotene protect your cells from free radicals either directly, by quenching them, or indirectly, by helping create the enzymes that quench them. Vitamin E is particularly helpful for protecting your cell membranes. Vitamin C is a potent antioxidant, and because it's water-soluble, it can go everywhere inside and outside your cells. But don't let me get ahead of myself.

You'll be reading about all the antioxidant vitanutrients in Chapters 8 and 9.

Many compounds found naturally in plant foods are extremely valuable for quenching the free radicals that are produced when your liver removes toxins and wastes from your body. The sulforaphane found so abundantly in broccoli, cauliflower, and other cruciferous vegetables, for instance, is very effective. So is the genistein found in soy foods and the polyphenols found in red wine, tea, and many other foods. Foods that are high in phytic acid, such as whole grains, are natural chelating agents that help remove trace minerals that could trigger free radical reactions. You'll read more about how these compounds work, and which ones work best, in later chapters.

Because enzymes are proteins, you also need amino acids, the building blocks of proteins, to make them. You can't make glutathione, for example, without N-acetyl cysteine (NAC), a form of the amino acid cysteine. Nor can you make antioxidant enzymes without a good supply of trace minerals. Selenium is one example. You need it to make glutathione; not enough selenium, not enough glutathione. Likewise, you need iron to make catalase, and you need zinc, copper, and manganese to make SOD.

Eating all the good foods in the world won't help your antioxidant levels if you're also taking drugs that suppress them. There's a very long list of drugs that deplete the trace minerals and vitamins you need to manufacture antioxidant enzymes. Some of the more obvious culprits are well-known to you, I'm sure. Over-the-counter medications H_2 blockers [Tagamet, Zantac, and the antihistamine pseudoephedrine (Sudafed)] block your use of antioxidants and let the free radicals run wild. Broad-spectrum prescription antibiotics also have a negative effect on your antioxidant level. Worst of all by far are the dangerous corticosteroids. If you're on a cortisone drug such as prednisone, make sure you check out Chapter 13 on natural hormones to understand the reasons not to take it and to find helpful ways to get off it.

DIETS AND SUPPLEMENTS

Later chapters of this book will specify the antioxidant vitanutrients and foods you should be consuming to reduce free radical damage and the aging it causes. For now, just remember that a good supply of vitanutrients is essential to produce the antioxidant enzymes you need to live a longer, healthier life.

Let me return to Dr. Harman for more on the subject. In 1999, he wrote that "the increases in the percentage of elderly people in the population since 1960 and the declining incidence of chronic disability among them, decreases in cancer mortality since 1991, and continuing declines in cardiovascular disease are in accord with the beneficial effects expected from the growing use of antioxidant supplements since the 1960s . . . as well as the growing publicity about the ability of fruits and vegetables to decrease disease incidence by depressing free radical reaction damage."[5]

Note carefully what Dr. Harman is saying here. The advances in longevity and health in the past few decades are due more to diet and vitanutrients than to anything the medical establishment has done. I heartily concur. But before I take up the specific techniques I and my

colleagues use to keep people healthy—and long-lived—
I need to touch on a particularly pernicious antiaging
theory, the caloric restriction road to long life, and to
tell you why it's bunk.

7

CALORIC RESTRICTION—AND WHY YOU SHOULDN'T DO IT

No discussion of antiaging theories can be complete without telling you about one of the best-researched and most generously documented theories of how to extend your life span: the concept of restricting total caloric intake.

Caloric restriction means a diet that's low in calories while still containing all the essential nutrients. As defined by its "inventor," UCLA researcher and Biospherean Roy Walford, it's "undernutrition without malnutrition."[1] Walford's theory is that if you eat fewer calories, you'll burn less oxygen in your mitochondria, which in turn means you'll produce fewer free radicals. The theory is obviously closely tied to Denham Harman's conclusion that the accumulation of free radicals is the major cause of aging. Caloric restriction thus becomes a way of stopping free radical production at the source.

If you've read any of my other books, you know that my very successful approach to weight loss is based on the idea that caloric restriction is an unacceptable activity. But in truth, even when caloric restriction is aimed not at weight loss but at extending life span, as it is in Walford's theory, I still think it's a terrible idea. I'm inclined to agree with the individual who opined, when hearing about this not-very-thrilling option: "You may not live to be one hundred, but you'll be hungry enough that it'll sure *seem* like it."

Nevertheless, precisely because of all the research and documentation—not to mention all the publicity—caloric restriction deserves our attention, as does the argument against it.

OF MICE AND MONKEYS

I've never seen an antiaging theory so well documented by studies on lab rodents. All the studies show that caloric restriction—sometimes cutting animals' food consumption by more than half their normal intake—significantly extends their life spans. On average, lab rats and mice that are restricted to only 60 to 70 percent of the amount that control rats eat live 25 percent, 40 percent, even 50 percent longer.[2] They also appear younger and healthier for longer, with fewer tumors and higher levels of disease-fighting white blood cells.

In fact, caloric restriction is the *only* thing that has been proven to extend the life span of experimental animals. People aren't lab rats, of course, so it's not clear if caloric restriction would really extend a human's life span.

Humans and monkeys, however, are a lot closer relatives, and caloric restriction studies on monkeys are producing results similar to those with rats. The calorically restricted monkeys are healthier and more youthful-looking than those on the regular diet. They're also a lot hungrier. But since monkeys live on average about twenty to thirty years, it's far too soon to say if caloric restriction will actually extend their lives.

Another factor to consider is that what applies to the diets of rats and monkeys in laboratory conditions doesn't have much application to the diets of humans in the real world. Also, it's easy to design a standard diet, calorically restricted or otherwise, for lab animals that have been bred for decades for uniformity and live in carefully controlled lab conditions. It's much, much harder to come up with a standard diet that's good for all humans, with our infinite variability in size, metabolism, genetic makeup, and activity level. For those reasons, I find the animal evidence on caloric restriction less than convincing for human application.

Besides, despite a lot of hungry rats, no one has yet shown exactly why caloric restriction extends life spans or how it works. There's no proof that it works by reducing the animals' lifetime production of free radicals, although many researchers *believe* that's the underlying reason.

Recently, in fact, other researchers have suggested that the real benefit of caloric restriction comes simply from a reduction in body fat, which in turn decreases the amount of the various hormones and other chemical messengers body fat secretes.[3] Since many of those substances play a role in causing such health problems as insulin resistance, what all the caloric restriction experiment may be proving is something we've known for a long time: Being normal weight is healthier in general than being overweight, even if you're a lab animal.

On the other hand, calorically restricted rats have higher levels of stress hormones. If you've ever gone on the sort of low-calorie diet recommended by the medical establishment, you can understand why. The stress doesn't seem to be so severe that it hurts the rats, but nobody really knows. Maybe if the rats got somewhat more food, they'd produce fewer stress hormones and do equally well.

HUNGRY HUMANS

The only human study of caloric restriction happened by accident. It was about a year into the Biosphere 2 experiment, a two-year attempt to live in a closed, self-sustaining environment. That's when it became clear that the Biosphere 2 residents couldn't raise enough food to feed themselves the 2,500 calories a day considered necessary to individuals in good health who lead physically active lives. Roy Walford took advantage of the situation to put all the Biosphereans on an 1,800-calorie-per-day diet, along with vitamin and mineral supplements. The experiment lasted only a limited time, during which the food supplies had to be locked away to keep the crew from cheating. All the participants lost weight, to be sure—even Walford, very lean to begin with, lost twenty pounds—and their blood glucose, cholesterol, and blood pressure went down. Of course, those results could also have been due to the vigorous, persistent physical activity required to sustain daily life in Biosphere 2.

Besides, is leaner healthier? Not necessarily. Statistical evidence from the ongoing Nurses' Health Study of more than 100,000 women shows that the difference in death rates between lean and plump women of the same height and age was negligible. Only the obese women—women 20 percent or more over their ideal weights—had a significantly higher risk of death.[4]

So far as I know, one 1,800-calorie-per-day experiment was enough for all the researchers except Walford, who continues to "experiment" with antiaging caloric restriction on himself. None of the other calorie restricters became apostles for the theory. In fact, one reason there's been only one human study of caloric restriction—and that one by accident—is that the crew members participating in the experiment were in a setting much like a laboratory, and they were committed to staying there, hungry or not. I seriously doubt that anyone could stick to this sort of diet for very long in normal circumstances, no matter how much longer it might help you live. It certainly isn't much of a normal life—you're a little hungry all the time, as Roy Walford himself admits in interviews. I suspect that the species *Homo sapiens* is too sapient to fall for a lifetime of going hungry.

DIETING WITHOUT HUNGER

Do you have to walk around starved to be at your normal weight? Of course not, as anyone who's ever read one of my other books already knows. There's an easy, realistic way to get the main benefits of caloric restriction without going hungry and counting the minutes till your next meager rations. In fact, the one way to go through life eating fewer calories and *not* being constantly hungry is to significantly restrict the carbohydrates in your diet.

This fact was originally brought home to me in a crucial research paper, written in 1963 by Dr. Walter Lyons Bloom and Dr. Gordon Azar, that described the similarity between carbohydrate restriction—*not* caloric restriction—and fasting.[5]

The premise for the research was the observation that after two days of fasting, people feel very little hunger. What the Bloom-Azar study showed was that the same lack of hunger could be achieved merely by eliminating carbohydrates from the diet. Why? Because your body can store only a few thousand calories of carbohydrate as glycogen. When that gets used up, your body automatically switches over to burning your stored fat. All the fat-mobilizing catalysts, enzymes, and hormones your body puts out when the switch takes place combine to cut down your appetite.

It's possible that calorically restricted lab rats might do just as well if they were given a low-carbohydrate rat chow instead of just less of their regular rat chow. I've searched the scientific literature and haven't found a single study taking this approach. I wish some research institute would, because I know of millions of people who would be happy to go through life eating steak, lobster, chicken, cheese, eggs, and other luxurious, satisfying foods along with plenty of salad and fresh vegetables. If we could show that this approach works in rats, then a lot of people would beg to be among the volunteers studying whether it extends the human life span. At the least, the people who followed my approach would find themselves living out their full life expectancies instead of shortening them with a high-carbohydrate eating pattern.

To lose weight or even keep yourself at your current healthy weight, you don't need to count calories, much less restrict them. By eating intelligently based on the information in this book, you'll fill up quickly on tasty, satisfying, and nutrient-dense food. You won't feel the need to stuff yourself with carbohydrate-laden junk. If you bothered to count, you might find that you were eating somewhat fewer calories, but that doesn't matter. It's the quality of your calories, not the number of them, that makes the difference.

Calories—or the lack of them—are not the only thing that will help you defy aging. A wide range of antioxidant supplements, including vitamins, minerals, and many other vitanutrients, give you extra protection from free radicals. These vitanutrients are so valuable as age-defying substances that they form an essential part of the program I'm offering in this book.

It's now time to turn to them.

8

ANTIOXIDANTS ARE "VITAL" NUTRIENTS

Nutrition dominates the *Age-Defying Diet*—nutrition in the food you eat and extra nutrition through vitanutrient supplements. And central to nutrition are the antioxidants that neutralize free radical damage.

But it isn't only for their age-antidote capacity that I stress antioxidants in food and supplements. They also go beyond the free-radical battle to help us in many ways. When you make antioxidants part of an overall plan of diet and vitanutrients, you're improving your overall health as well as sending them out to fight the effects of aging.

And fight they will. The role of such antioxidant vitanutrients as vitamin C and E in enhancing your health and longevity has been so well established that it's astonishing to me that there could still be a question about them in the mind of any physician. Over the past few years, major articles about the benefits of antioxidant vitamins have appeared even in those fortresses of the medical establishment, *The New England Journal of Medicine* and the *Journal of the American Medical Association.*

To take just one example: A 1995 study reported in *JAMA* showed that antioxidant vitamins could slow the progression of coronary artery disease by slowing plaque buildup. The vitamins work by preventing free radical damage to the LDL cholesterol in the blood.[1] You couldn't ask for better evidence—and it was published in the house organ of what I believe is the most anti-nutrition force in medicine, the AMA.

Likewise, study after study has proven that vitamin E is a significant antioxidant that fights off atherosclerosis, protects your eyesight, and prevents cancer. Yet despite this clear and convincing evidence about vitamin E's life-or-death importance to your health, your conventional doctor may not suggest taking it—even though he's likely to be taking it himself. Why does someone pledged to preserving the health of patients deprive them of such a valuable vitanutrient?

Among other reasons, it's because the American Heart Association continues to withhold its seal of approval from vitanutrients. Here's what the AHA tells physicians and the public: "Although diet alone may not provide the levels of Vitamin E intake that have been associated with lowest risk in a few observational studies, the absence of efficacy and safety data from randomized trials precludes the establishment of population-wide recommendations regarding Vitamin E supplementation."[2]

This is typical of mainstream medicine's love affair with proof. Absolute proof, however, is not easy to establish. Whenever I meet proof-worshipers, I ask if they love their parents or their spouse. They always answer, "Certainly." My response to that: "Okay, prove it." In both areas—love and medicine—I prefer to rely on the best available evidence.

Despite the very powerful evidence in favor of antioxidant vitanutrients, however, and even though it's been repeatedly presented in the journals that every physician reads and relies on, your doctor probably won't tell you anything about how antioxidant vitanutrients can prevent free radical damage.

That's my job.

In this chapter, we'll look at the major circulating antioxidant vitamins and minerals: vitamins E and C, lipoic acid, and selenium. We'll learn how they work—individually and as a team—and we'll see what they do to improve our health and extend our lives. In the chapters that follow, we'll look more closely at the antioxidant enzymes, the carotenoids, and the bioflavonoids. By the time you're ready to move on to the techniques to defy aging, you'll have a good grasp of the powerful role these valuable vitanutrients can play in your life.

YOUR PRIME ANTIOXIDANTS

Vitamin E, vitamin C, lipoic acid, and selenium are the substances your body needs to mount its primary defense against free radicals, to say nothing of all the other important things they do for you.* All are essential elements in the antioxidant enzymes superoxide dismutase (SOD), catalase, and glutathione—enzymes your cells make to neutralize free radicals. If you don't have enough of the right vitamins and minerals to go around, you can't make enough of the enzymes—and the free radicals get the upper hand. When they do, it can lead to heart disease, stroke, cancer, and memory loss and other cognitive problems.

High levels of these prime antioxidants are thus essential to fight those diseases. They also protect against inflammatory arthritis[3] and sight-robbing cataracts and

*For detailed information, please see *Dr. Atkins' Vita-Nutrient Solution.*

macular degeneration. And of course, they counteract the free radical cause of aging itself.

Let's look at how each of them operates.

ACTIONS AND INTERACTIONS

Vitamin E is fat-soluble, which means it's especially good at entering your cell membranes and protecting them from free radical damage, especially from peroxyl radicals. Just as important, vitamin E keeps the tiny droplets of the bad LDL cholesterol in your blood from being oxidized. When any of the fats in your body, including cholesterol, get attacked by free radicals, they combine with oxygen, that is, they oxidize. The process is exactly the same as the one that makes butter go rancid. In effect, so is the result. You definitely want to do everything you can to keep your LDL cholesterol from oxidizing.

Vitamin C is water-soluble, which means it's found in all the water-bearing parts of your body—inside your cells, in the spaces in between your cells, in your blood, and in all the other fluids your body makes.

Lipoic acid (also called alpha lipoic acid or thioctic acid) is both fat-soluble *and* water-soluble; that makes it a universal antioxidant that's found in all the tissues of your body.

Lipoic acid has two main functions in your body. First, it's an essential co-factor for energy production in the mitochondria, and you'll remember from the previous chapter how extremely important mitochondria are to the aging process. Without lipoic acid, you can't make the enzymes that convert glucose and fatty acids into energy. In fact, lipoic acid is so important to your metabolism that when it was first isolated in the 1950s, researchers initially thought it was a vitamin. It's not, although it's certainly a vitanutrient.

As it turns out, however, your body manufactures only very, very limited amounts of lipoic acid, most of which becomes tightly attached to the enzymes in your mitochondria. It's only what's left over from that function that serves as such a powerful antioxidant, sponging up free radicals of all sorts. The leftovers available, unfortunately, constitute a really small amount, so to get the full benefit of lipoic acid, you'll need supplements.

Vitamin E, vitamin C, and lipoic acid are all valuable on their own, but as a team they're even better. That's because whenever a molecule of vitamin E or vitamin C neutralizes a free radical, the vitamin molecule itself becomes a free radical—although one that's far less dangerous. In a complex cycle, vitamin C, vitamin E, and lipoic acid interact with each other to regenerate the vitamins, which extends their useful life in your body and lets them get back to work. In other words, no one of these prime antioxidants is a miracle cure for all your ills. To maintain good health, you need them all, plus one more: selenium.

A trace mineral required in only minute amounts, selenium is a crucial ingredient for supporting the activity of vitamin E and for making glutathione peroxidase, your body's most abundant antioxidant enzyme. Glutathione is also involved in the vitamin regeneration cycle, and both lipoic acid and selenium are essential ingredients for making it. In addition, all on its own, selenium has the best scientific claim to being called a powerful cancer-preventing vitanutrient.

What impact do the prime antioxidants have on aging? Let's put it all together and see how they work—both individually and as a team—to protect your health as you get older.

PREVENTING HEART DISEASE

There's no question that high levels of antioxidant vitamins prevent or slow heart disease. The evidence is very powerful for three of our four prime antioxidants.

Vitamin E

Here's just some of the proof that continues to pile up about vitamin E's role in preventing heart disease:

- The long-running, Harvard-based Physicians' Health Study showed in 1993 that men who take just 100 International Units, or IU, of vitamin E daily have nearly half the risk of coronary artery disease as men who get less than 7 IU daily.[4]
- The equally long-running Nurses' Health Study showed in 1993 that women who took vitamin E supplements for two years cut their risk of coronary artery disease in half compared to women who didn't take the supplements.[5]
- The well-known Cambridge Heart Antioxidant Study (CHAOS) looked at 40,000 men who already had heart disease. The study found that vitamin E kept the disease from getting worse. The men who took at least 400 IU of vitamin E a day cut their risk of a nonfatal heart attack by an amazing 77 percent.[6]
- A 1996 study from the University of California School of Medicine showed that taking 100 IU of vitamin E a day substantially slowed the progress of coronary artery disease in men who already had it.[7]
- A long-term study of postmenopausal women

showed that those who ate the most foods high in vitamin E—for example, nuts, vegetable oils, and avocado—had strikingly less heart disease. That's without taking vitamin E supplements.[8]

In addition to these revealing studies, some very recent research suggests that vitamin E also reduces the activity of a blood enzyme that plays a role in plaque formation. Vitamin E breaks the chemical chain and prevents the reaction that triggers plaque.[9]

It also makes your blood "thinner" in general, so it's less likely to clot where you don't want it—for example, in an artery leading to your heart or brain. In fact, vitamin E works almost as well as the anticoagulating drug warfarin (Coumadin) but in a different way: It prevents the tiny blood-clotting particles called platelets from clumping together. Of course, it costs a lot less and it's a lot safer, which may be why the medical-pharmaceutical complex keeps mum about its capabilities. (Actually, I dislike the misleading term "blood thinner." The appropriate term is "anticoagulant," something that keeps your blood from clotting. Vitamin E works so well to reduce your blood's ability to clot that you're advised to stop taking it for a couple of weeks before any scheduled surgery.)

Vitamin C

Now, what about vitamin C? The evidence here is also very solid. For example, a recent piece of research showed that if your blood levels of vitamin C are low to the point of being deficient, your risk of a heart attack is about 3.5 times greater than for someone with a normal blood level of vitamin C.[10]

And you'd be surprised how many people are in fact deficient in vitamin C, despite living in an era of fortified foods. Studies show that some 25 percent of older men have low serum levels,[11] while overall, about 30 percent of the adult population is low on vitamin C, and more than 6 percent are outright deficient.[12] All these people are at greater risk for heart disease—as well as for cancer, cataracts, and other problems that could be prevented by simple, safe, and very inexpensive vitamin supplements.

If you already have atherosclerosis, your chances of having a heart attack or an episode of unstable angina are much higher if you're low on vitamin C. The vitamin C doesn't do anything to reduce the size of plaques, but it does keep them from rupturing and causing a blockage in the artery.[13]

The powerful evidence for vitamin C's efficacy makes it particularly unfortunate that this vitanutrient is plagued by a terrible misconception. In 1998, researchers reported that high doses of vitamin C seemed actually to cause free radical damage to the DNA in your cells. The anti-vitamin medical establishment and the media seized on this opportunity to undermine vitamin C. They took a single, very short research letter with very tentative conclusions—not a full-fledged, peer-reviewed scientific study—and made it sound as if taking a vitamin C supplement could turn you into some sort of genetically mutated monster.[14]

What the media reports didn't tell you is that even an ordinary celery stalk contains compounds that can damage DNA. The media also didn't tell you that *too little* vitamin C is well documented as a potential cause of DNA damage.[15] That knowledge should get you to ask the critics, "With regard to protecting DNA, what is the optimal range of vitamin C?" I don't know what they'll say, but I know what I would say: "The optimal range is whatever it was before that research letter was published."

Let me assure you that this one single report is no reason to stop taking vitamin C. Its questionable conclusion is outweighed many times over by the numerous studies that prove vitamin C's value as a safe, powerful, and very effective antioxidant.

Selenium

Selenium's role in preventing heart disease is sometimes overlooked. In fact, low selenium levels, like low vitamin C levels, are a serious risk factor for heart disease.[16] If you're low on selenium, you're going to be low on glutathione as well, and that means that your antioxidant defenses really are dangerously low.

In addition to its role in making glutathione, selenium helps your heart by removing such dangerous heavy metals as mercury and lead. These minerals are bad for you in general, but they're especially damaging to your heart tissues.

PROTECTING YOUR BRAIN

Your brain has literally trillions of closely packed cells that communicate with each other across cell membranes. Free radicals attack the membranes and damage the lines of communication, closing them down. To keep the lines open and static-free, you need to protect your brain cells against free radical damage. The best protection you can give is a high antioxidant level. Huge amounts of research have been carried out in this area, and an awful lot of it points to antioxidants as a valuable way to prevent memory loss, Alzheimer's disease, and other cognition problems related to aging.

- In a recent study of retired people in Australia, the ones who took vitamin C supplements showed significantly less cognitive impairment, as much as 60 percent less. When the researchers added dietary vitamin C, the decrease in impairment jumped to almost 70 percent.[17] I'm not surprised by this—your vitamin C levels are ten times higher in your brain than they are elsewhere in your body. Keeping that level high, as it's meant to be, is the most natural approach to keeping your brain working well.

- The antioxidant power of vitamin E can keep you from having a brain-destroying stroke. Researchers at Columbia-Presbyterian Hospital in New York City showed in 1999 that even small amounts of supplemental vitamin E protect you against an ischemic stroke—a stroke caused by a blood clot or arterial disease blocking the flow of blood to the brain. According to this study, vitamin E supplements cut your risk of ischemic stroke by 53 percent.[18]

- A high intake of vitamin E can help ward off the annoying memory problems associated with aging. In a study of healthy older people age fifty to seventy-five, the people with the highest blood level of vitamin E did best on tests of memory. Why? Because vitamin E protects your brain cells—which are particularly high in fat— against the damaging effects of free radicals.[19]

- Vitamin E was just as effective as the drug selegiline in significantly slowing the progression of Alzheimer's disease—without the major expense of the drug.[20]

- Lipoic acid may play a part in preventing the cell damage that causes Alzheimer's disease, and it may also help slow the damage if it does start. The research here is very promising.[21]

In addition to the power of antioxidants to keep blood flowing smoothly to your brain, other vitanutrients, such as ginkgo biloba, are extremely valuable for cerebral circulation. I'll get to them later on, in Chapter 18.

PREVENTING CANCER

I have emphasized how valuable the eradication of cardiovascular disease is in extending your life span. There's another illness whose eradication would be just as welcome in the fight against aging: cancer.

Your chances of getting cancer go up as you age. Is that something you just have to accept? Absolutely not. You can take all sorts of positive steps to prevent cancer through vitanutrients. Indeed, vitamin C is proving to be one of the most powerful anticarcinogenic agents of all.[22]

I could write a whole book just discussing the many studies that prove the value of vitamin C against cancer. Here's the gist of it: Vitamin C sharply reduces your chances of getting cancer of the stomach, esophagus, colon, bladder, cervix, uterus, and breast.[23] It probably helps prevent many other cancers as well, but the evidence has yet to be made as clear-cut.

But prevention isn't the whole story; vitamin C also plays a role in cancer treatment—a major role, in fact, according to alternative cancer therapists. At international meetings on alternative cancer treatments, research papers on the intravenous administration of vitamin C are generating great excitement. The papers report profound and immediate shrinkage of tumors. In addition, IV vitamin C is certainly a far safer approach to cancer than the traditional slash-and-burn, kill-everything approach of chemotherapy and radiation treatment. It's certainly far easier on the patient's health—and on his or her wallet. Even in large intravenous doses, vitamin C is inexpensive and easy to administer, with very few side effects.

Vitamin E also offers powerful cancer protection. Hundreds of positive studies have shown that overall, the more vitamin E you get, the lower your chances of getting any sort of cancer. Just consider the recent results from an ongoing research project called the Alpha-Tocopherol, Beta-Carotene Cancer Prevention Study (the ABC study for short). In 1998, the ABC study showed that vitamin E supplementation can protect against prostate cancer. The study showed that men over fifty who take just 50 IU of supplemental vitamin E have a 36 percent lower incidence of prostate cancer. It showed that among men who do get prostate cancer, taking vitamin E cuts their chance of dying from the disease by 41 percent.[24] Bear in mind that there are about 100,000 new cases of prostate cancer in the United States each year. Reducing its incidence by almost a third through a vitanutrient that costs just a few pennies a day would have a major impact on national health care costs. (Another vitanutrient, called lycopene, also protects against prostate cancer. I'll discuss it in depth in Chapter 10.)

Alternative practitioners like myself have known for a long time that the trace mineral selenium also helps prevent cancer. Our belief was vindicated by the results of a major study published in 1997. The researchers already knew from earlier studies that people with low blood levels of selenium have a higher likelihood of developing skin cancer. They also knew that people who live in areas where diets are naturally rich in selenium are less likely to die of cancer than are people who live in areas where dietary selenium is low. Putting these facts together, the researchers reasoned that giving selenium supplements to people who already had skin cancer could prevent a recurrence.

It didn't. More than 1,300 patients participated in the study, with half taking daily supplements of 200 mcg of selenium and half taking a placebo. At the end of the ten-year study, the number of new skin cancers was the same in both groups. But the patients who took selenium supplements had sharply lowered rates of *other* cancers: 63 percent fewer prostate cancers, 67 percent fewer esophageal cancers, 58 percent fewer colorectal cancers, and 46 percent fewer lung cancers. Overall, the selenium supplements reduced the number of cancers in the group by a third and cut cancer deaths in half.[25]

The results of this important study were published in the prestigious *Journal of the American Medical Association*. An accompanying editorial was headlined "Selenium and cancer prevention: Promising results indicate further trials required"—the typical response of the medical mainstream to any therapy that smacks of being "alternative." As usual with any vitanutrient approach to illness, the AMA refuses to make a recommendation and instead insists that more study is needed, no matter how many lives could be extended.[26]

But even the AMA can't ignore the results of the ongoing research on selenium forever. Since the 1997 study editorialized about in *JAMA*, the protective effect of selenium against cancer has been reconfirmed by a number of other studies. To take just one example, a study of more than 33,000 men showed that selenium significantly reduces the risk of prostate cancer. Among study participants who took 200 mcg of selenium every day for five years, the risk of prostate cancer was one-third that of men who took a placebo instead.[27] I'll let that powerful evidence speak for itself.

One more word on the ability of antioxidants to fight cancer: They work most powerfully when they work as a team with other vitanutrients. Atkins Center patients at risk for a recurrence of cancer are routinely given an entire battery of antioxidants. In addition to the four prime antioxidants, they are routinely prescribed mixed carotenoids—including natural beta-carotene and lyco-pene—such flavonoids as quercetin and proanthocyani-dins, coenzyme Q_{10}, and glutathione builders like N-acetyl cysteine. (I'll talk more about all these supplements in the next couple of chapters.) All our doctors are convinced that our recurrence rate is dramatically lower than that achieved by those treated in the conventional way with chemotherapy and/or radiation.

SAVING YOUR SIGHT WITH ANTIOXIDANTS

The delicate structures of your eyes are particularly vulnerable to free radical damage, mostly because your eyes are exposed to a lot of ultraviolet light. The older you get, the more the damage and the higher your risk of sight-robbing cataracts and macular degeneration. But high levels of vitamin C and vitamin E can do a lot to prevent these problems.

In fact, taking vitamin E supplements could cut your risk of a cataract by half.[28] Even a regular one-a-day multivitamin supplement that contains only small amounts of vitamin E cuts your chances of a cataract by about 25 percent.[29]

If you think that's impressive, look at the statistics for

vitamin C. Taking vitamin C supplements on a long-term basis could cut your risk of a cataract by 77 percent; that's the conclusion from a 1997 study of women who had been taking extra C for ten years or more.[30] Given that about 12 percent of the annual Medicare budget goes for cataract surgery, the study would seem to argue convincingly that taking vitanutrients saves not just your health but also your money.

Antioxidant vitamins and other antioxidant nutrients are also crucial for preventing macular degeneration, the leading cause of blindness among adults over fifty. Current projections are for some 6.3 million cases of macular degeneration among older Americans by 2030. As I'll explain in the next chapter, many of these cases could be prevented by taking vitamin C and vitamin E along with supplements containing such carotenoids as lutein and zeaxanthin. Of course, eating plenty of the foods that contain these substances naturally—including dark-green leafy vegetables like kale—will also help.

IMMUNITY AND ANTIOXIDANTS

As you've gotten older, you may have noticed that minor illnesses you once shook off easily now stay with you longer. The cold that barely slowed you down when you were twenty puts you to bed for a week at age fifty. That's because reduced immunity is part of the aging process. As with all the effects of aging, it can be fought.

Few weapons are as powerful as vitanutrients in the battle to keep your immune system functioning at peak capacity. Building up your immunity is so important for your ongoing health and longevity that I've given it a chapter of its own (Chapter 15). I mention it here to let you know that antioxidants cover the immunity base as well as all the others I've been discussing, but for a comprehensive discussion of the issue, please hold on.

CHOOSING YOUR ANTIOXIDANT SUPPLEMENTS

Now that you know what antioxidants can do to fight disease, you're probably asking how to choose your supplements and how much you should take. Let's deal with dosage first.

In general, you'll need fairly high amounts to get the full protective effect. The benefits of vitamin E, for instance, show up only in daily doses of at least 50 IU; bigger doses—at least 400 IU daily—are preferable. There's no reasonable way you can eat enough foods high in vitamin E to get those amounts. Even a typical daily multivitamin supplement only has 30 IU of vitamin E. To get anywhere near levels that would do you some good, you'll have to take supplements.

As to the safety issue, vitamin E supplements even in very large doses of over 2,000 IU daily are perfectly safe for just about everybody. In fact, I put virtually every patient at the Atkins Center on large, safe doses of vitamin E.

In choosing your vitamin E supplements, it's helpful to know that vitamin E is really a catch-all name for a group of related compounds that work together to protect you from free radicals. These include two main types of active ingredients: tocopherols and tocotrienols. To simplify some complex chemistry, the tocopherol portion of vitamin E has four components: alpha-, beta-, gamma-, and delta-tocopherol. Of these four, alpha-tocopherol is the most active. It's the one that works hardest to destroy free radicals, and it's the one most easily handled by your liver, the place where vitamin E is metabolized. The other tocopherols also play a part, even though they're less active. Look for a vitamin E supplement that contains natural mixed tocopherols. That's the way vitamin E appears in nature, which means that's the way your body is designed to absorb it.

Like the tocopherols, the tocotrienols also come in alpha, beta, gamma, and delta versions. There's some good evidence to show that the tocotrienols are valuable for free radical protection, especially from the peroxyl radical. Unfortunately, tocotrienol supplements are very expensive. If you want to spend the money, look for vitamin E supplements that have mixed tocopherols and tocotrienols.

Whatever form you choose, to get the maximum benefit from your vitamin E capsules, take them with a meal. The fat in your food helps your body absorb the vitamin.

Today many manufacturers make vitamin E capsules with added selenium. This is a good, convenient way to be sure you're getting the best of both vitanutrients. In general, you need about 400 mcg of selenium a day to get the maximum protection. People have been warned against taking much more than that—doses higher than 1,000 mcg (1 mg) could be toxic over a long period. But whenever selenium is necessary to reverse an illness, I don't hesitate to give double the dose during the first few months.

Given that the recommended daily allowance (RDA) for vitamin C is a ridiculously low 60 mg, you might not think that anyone could really be deficient. (The RDA will probably be raised to between 100 and 200 mg in the near future—an improvement, but still far too low.) In fact, about a quarter of all Americans get less than 40 mg a day from their food.[31] There is no better, cheaper, more effective way to prevent all the health problems I've discussed in this chapter than to give everyone the optimal dose of vitamin C every day. What would that be? My usual recommended range is 800 to 2,000 mg daily.

Because vitamin C is water-soluble, spread your dose out over the day. Taking it all at once will lead to a lot of excretion from your body. Try to get as much vitamin C as possible from your food as well.

Lipoic acid is another extremely safe vitanutrient. I usually recommend between 200 and 400 mg a day, more if the patient already has diabetes. That's because lipoic acid is a very effective treatment for diabetes, especially diabetic neuropathy.

The prime antioxidant vitamins and minerals are your first line of defense against free radical damage. They're also essential for making the antioxidant enzymes that are your body's other major defense system. Let's turn to those next.

9

THE ANTIOXIDANT ENZYMES

Humans are among the most long-lived of animals; only some kinds of turtles and perhaps a few whales outlive us. Humans also have levels of antioxidant enzymes higher than just about any other animals. Long life and high levels of antioxidant enzymes—it's not coincidence. The antioxidant enzymes are a powerful force for longevity. In this chapter, we'll learn what they are, how they work, and how they're made. We'll also explore how to raise your enzyme levels. And we'll look at a couple of the most promising "new" antioxidants that keep us from getting old: coenzyme Q_{10} and melatonin.

SOD, CATALASE, AND GLUTATHIONE

These are the big three antioxidant enzymes forming your body's own set of very powerful defenses against free radicals. You make all these enzymes right inside your cells all the time—they're exactly where they need to be in order to quench free radicals as soon as they're produced. Imagine the three as warriors in combat. Then think of SOD and catalase working hand in hand to quickly disarm the most dangerous free radicals, while glutathione does rear-guard mopping-up duty. Here's how it works.

When normal metabolism inside your mitochondria makes superoxide free radicals, SOD quickly converts them into oxygen and hydrogen peroxide. The only problem is that when a superoxide free radical meets hydrogen peroxide, it forms the very reactive free radical known as hydroxyl. Of all the free radicals, hydroxyl is the biggest vandal, the one that does the most damage in your body. You need to quench it instantly, just as soon as it's produced. Unfortunately, your body doesn't make an enzyme that can quench the hydroxyl radical (although, as I'll discuss later in this chapter, you do have other defenses). That's where catalase comes in. Catalase grabs the hydrogen peroxide and breaks it up into oxygen and water before it can form a hydroxyl radical. The oxygen and water then get reused by your cells as part of normal metabolism.

Catalase has one big limitation: It works only in the watery parts of your cells. It can't protect the fatty parts of a cell, like the cell membrane, from lipid peroxides— the free radicals that are formed when hydrogen peroxide attacks lipids.

That's where glutathione comes in. Glutathione is the most abundant antioxidant enzyme in your body. It's everywhere, both inside and outside your cells. In the form of glutathione peroxidase, it patrols your cells looking for any molecules of hydrogen peroxide your catalase has missed. It also protects your cell membranes against lipid peroxidation, a process that kicks in whenever any free radical steals an electron from the delicate fatty membrane of a cell. Lipid peroxidation, like all free radical damage, is a chain reaction that keeps going until something puts a stop to it—in this case, glutathione peroxidase. Without the glutathione, the damage would continue, and the cell membrane would grow weaker and weaker until finally the cell was irretrievably damaged and died. If the lipid peroxides are quenched quickly, however, your body can repair the cell membrane and get things working properly again.

Glutathione peroxidase is continually recycled in your body through a complicated set of chemical reactions with the other forms of glutathione—glutathione reductase and glutathione transferase. (Glutathione also plays an important role in your liver as part of the process for removing toxins. I'll explain more about that in Chapter 16 on detoxification.)

RAISING YOUR ENZYME LEVELS

Since your antioxidant enzymes are manufactured inside your cells by your body as you need them, is there anything you can do to raise their levels? Yes, at least to some degree.

You probably remember from high school biology that an enzyme is a protein your body manufactures in order to speed up the various biochemical processes of your metabolism. What's interesting about enzymes is that a little goes a long way—small amounts have big effects. The other side of that, though, is that you need every little bit. Being even a little low on the antioxidant enzymes can have serious consequences.

Like all the proteins in your body, enzymes are assembled in your cells from building blocks called amino acids, according to instructions handed down by the DNA in the nucleus of every cell. Vitamin C, the B vitamins, and trace amounts of some minerals—copper, zinc, manganese, and iron—are also needed to help the proteins fit together properly.

In fact, every time you need to manufacture an enzyme in your cells, *all* the raw materials and precisely the *right* raw materials need to be on hand. If even one minor ingredient isn't readily available, you either won't be able to make enough of the enzyme or you won't be able to make it fast enough. Picture an assembly line grinding to a halt because the wrong screw—or none at all—got fed into the supply chain; it's exactly the same thing. Starve your cells of what they need, and the enzymes won't be assembled quickly enough. Even worse, without a regular supply of essential ingredients, your antioxidant enzymes could get out of balance. If you make enough SOD but not enough catalase, for instance, the all-important balance between the two is thrown off. They won't be able to work in tandem to protect you. Only when you give your cells enough of all the right building blocks will they be able to put together the antioxidant enzymes as quickly as you need them.

THE AMINOS

Your body manufactures some 50,000 different proteins from just twenty-two amino acids, in the same way, in a sense, as we can write all the words of the English language using just twenty-six letters. These building blocks of protein fall into two categories: essential and nonessential. The nine essential amino acids are the ones you must get from food; the essentials are also the ingredients your body uses to put together the other thirteen nonessential aminos.

The nonessential aminos *may* occur in food, but our bodies can't get them from food. We can get them only when the essential aminos make them, and the essential aminos can make them only when our food contains enough of the essentials to build them. And even though they're called *non*essential, that doesn't mean we don't need them. We do. The bottom line, therefore, is that we must eat enough of the right foods to supply us with sufficient essential amino acids to meet our needs for the essential aminos on their own and for the nonessentials they make for us.

But when it comes to aminos, not all foods are equal. Only animal foods—meat, eggs, fish, and dairy products—contain all nine of the essential amino acids, along with varying amounts of other nonessential aminos. They're what nutritionists call high-quality or complete proteins. And of all these high-quality proteins, which one is the very best? If you've read my other books, you already know: the egg. In fact, the egg is the standard nutritionists use to measure the quality of other proteins.

Of course, eggs have been dubbed "nutritionally incorrect" by much of the medical profession. In fact, many of the patients who first come to me at the Atkins Center have eliminated eggs from their diet in the belief that they're doing something positive for their health. Nothing could be further from the truth. By denying themselves the ideal source of the essential amino acids they badly need, these patients are actually doing themselves harm. One of the first things I recommend to them is to start eating eggs again, at least two a day.

Without a good supply of the essential amino acids eggs possess in rich abundance, your body can't assemble the antioxidant enzymes you need. And getting the aminos in eggs is better and more efficient than getting them in supplements.

SOD and catalase, for instance, are very complicated proteins, made up of long strings of amino acids; the string that makes SOD has about 150 units, the string that makes catalase has over 500. Because SOD and catalase are so complicated, taking oral supplements is an inefficient way to boost your levels. The proteins are quickly broken down into their basic amino acids by your digestive system. (Several manufacturers do make SOD tablets, but they don't seem to raise SOD levels very well, and injectable SOD has not yet been legalized.)

Glutathione, on the other hand, is very simple. It's made up of just three amino acids, so glutathione supplements may be more available to your body. That's because glutathione is a tripeptide—a very short string of just three amino acids. The string is so small that it doesn't get broken down further by your digestive system so you can absorb it whole into your bloodstream.

An even better way to raise your glutathione level is to raise your level of cysteine, an amino acid that's fundamental to manufacturing glutathione. We know that your blood levels of glutathione change in direct proportion to the amount of cysteine in your diet. The more cysteine you get, the more glutathione you make. To directly raise my patients' glutathione levels, I usually give them supplements of N-acetyl-cysteine (NAC), because the acetylated form leads to a higher glutathione level. But what's one of the very best dietary sources of cysteine? You guessed it—eggs. There are 146 mg of cysteine in one egg, most of it in the yolk.

If eggs are such a good source of the essential amino acids, why does your conventional doctor tell you to eat them only occasionally? Because he or she thinks eggs raise your cholesterol level. As with so much of the other cholesterol misinformation you're given, this particular myth is the gospel as preached by the American Heart Association. The AHA says you should take in only 300 mg a day of dietary cholesterol. Since one egg has about 215 mg of cholesterol—more than most other foods have for the same number of calories—you obviously shouldn't eat eggs. Or so the AHA claims. But the truth is there's very little connection between the cholesterol you eat and the cholesterol in your blood. You're at far greater risk from the deadly trans fats found in all the heavily processed foods most people eat, including margarine.

I could cite dozens of studies that show the opposite of the AHA position: that eating eggs actually improves your blood cholesterol profile. Here's just one good example. In a 1994 study, twenty-four adults added two eggs a day to their usual diets for six weeks. At the end of the period, their total cholesterol levels had increased by 4 percent. Their all-important HDL levels, however, were up a very desirable 10 percent.[1]

I'm glad to say that some members of the conventional medical world are finally starting to think for themselves. In 1999, the National Institutes of Health, a pretty conventional bunch, funded a major study that showed that eating an egg a day does not increase the risk of heart disease or stroke for healthy adults.[2] I can only hope that this will prompt some conventional doctors finally to take off their blinders and start recommending eggs to their patients. They're a great food altogether and a superb source of the amino acids your body needs to make antioxidant enzymes.

MINERALS AND VITAMINS

Adequate supplies of the trace minerals zinc, manganese, copper, sulfur, and selenium are also essential in making the antioxidant enzymes. Manganese is particularly important for making SOD inside your mitochondria, where most of your free radicals are produced. Selenium and sulfur are critical for forming glutathione. So, in addition to making sure you're getting enough high-quality protein every day, you need to be sure you're getting enough of the important trace minerals. (I'll discuss exactly how much you need of the trace minerals later on in Chapter 21. For detailed information on each one, see *Dr. Atkins' Vita-Nutrient Solution*.)

Finally, you need a goodly supply of vitamins, especially C and the B complex, to make the antioxidant enzymes. Vitamin C stimulates your body to produce extra catalase, and without vitamin B_6 (pyridoxine), you can't make glutathione.

COENZYME Q_{10}

Of all the vitanutrients I recommend for my patients, coenzyme Q_{10} (also known as CoQ_{10}) is one of the most valuable. This essential vitanutrient is absolutely necessary for you to create energy in your mitochondria. No CoQ_{10}, no energy—it's as simple as that. CoQ_{10} is so important for your body that it's found in every single one of your cells. In fact, it's so widespread in your body that another name for it is ubiquinone, combining the Latin *ubi*, meaning "everywhere," and *quinone*, a natural chemical crucial to energy production.

When CoQ_{10} was discovered back in the late 1950s, researchers thought that its only function was helping in energy production. By the early 1960s, however, it was being used widely in Japan to treat congestive heart failure, and in the 1970s, Japanese researchers had learned ways to produce CoQ_{10} easily. That's when research into CoQ_{10} really took off. Fast-forward to the 1980s, by which time CoQ_{10} had become of the five top-selling drugs in Japan.

In the United States, however, the FDA has declared in its ignorance that CoQ_{10} is a dietary supplement with no real medical value. This means that despite its proven record for treating patients with cardiovascular disease, and despite its virtual absence of side effects, an American cardiologist is very unlikely ever to prescribe CoQ_{10} to a patient. Instead, you'll be bombarded with dangerous drugs that simply mask the symptoms of your heart disease.

Since I'm focusing on antioxidants in this chapter, I won't go into how CoQ_{10} can be a life-saver for people with congestive heart failure, or how it helps people with diabetes control their blood sugar, or how patients with chronic fatigue syndrome have made near miraculous recoveries when they start taking it. I won't even talk about how it may help to revitalize the immune systems of cancer patients.

Instead, let's look at how CoQ_{10} works in your body. CoQ_{10} is called a coenzyme because you need it to make at least three and possibly more of the enzymes involved in converting glucose and oxygen in your mitochondria into energy. Once the energy is created, CoQ_{10} also becomes part of the complex process of getting it out of your mitochondria and into the rest of your body.

CoQ_{10} also acts as an antioxidant inside your mitochondria, quenching superoxide radicals as they're formed.[3] Recent research, however, tells us that CoQ_{10} plays a bigger antioxidant role than we realized. Because CoQ_{10} is everywhere in your body, and because it moves easily into and through your fatty cell membranes, it also helps prevent damage to your cells from lipid peroxidation—those damaging free radical attacks on cell membranes. It also works synergistically with vitamin E, vitamin C, and lipoic acid to keep all those antioxidant vitanutrients working longer to protect you.[4]

You reach your peak production of CoQ_{10} at around age twenty. After that, your production gradually drops off; the drop picks up speed as you pass forty. By the time you're eighty, you're naturally making only about 60 percent of your peak levels. At any age, though, your doctor may artificially lower your CoQ_{10} production to far below the optimal level. How? By prescribing cholesterol-lowering statin drugs—lovastatin, simvastatin, and others. CoQ_{10} shares some of the same production pathways as cholesterol. When statin drugs block the production of cholesterol in your liver, they also block your production of CoQ_{10}.

When that happens, you—and especially your heart—are in trouble. Your heart, like other high-energy parts of your body, needs high concentrations of CoQ_{10}; in fact, the level of CoQ_{10} in your heart is twice that of other parts of your body. At the same time, CoQ_{10} is one of the most important antioxidants protecting your heart and arteries against atherosclerosis.[5] If you've ever wondered why many studies show that the death rate from heart attacks for people who take statin drugs is still high, it's probably because the statin has severely reduced their CoQ_{10}.

To raise your CoQ_{10} level, you could eat foods that are high in it, such as sardines or beef liver, but you'd have to consume an awful lot of them for a dietary approach to have any real effect. Supplements are the way to go, but they are far from cheap. One reason is that with each successive year, doctors keep learning that higher doses are more beneficial. By now the preventive dosage that I recommend is 50 to 100 mg daily. If you have any sort of health problem related to the heart, high blood pressure, metabolism, or energy level, you'll probably need closer to 200 to 300 mg a day.

MELATONIN: THE UNSUNG ANTIOXIDANT

Melatonin, a hormone that regulates your body's twenty-four-hour clock, has been in the news a lot lately. You've probably heard that it's a natural sleeping pill that can help reset the internal clock thrown off by jet lag or shift changes, that it can help boost your immune system, even that it helps prevent cancer.

What you may not know is that melatonin is also a very powerful antioxidant. Remember the dangerous hydroxyl radicals I mentioned earlier in the chapter? Your antioxidant enzymes can't quench hydroxyl radicals, but melatonin can. Not only that, melatonin can stimulate your body to produce more of the other antioxidant enzymes that are the main subject of this chapter.

As with a lot of other hormones, you naturally make less melatonin as you get older. By the time you're fifty, you're making just a fraction of the melatonin you made as a young teenager. That's one reason older people often have trouble falling asleep or staying asleep—without enough melatonin, their sleep-wake cycle gets skewed.

But making less melatonin as you get older has much more serious consequences for your health than just tossing and turning at night. Melatonin is extremely important for protecting your cells—especially your brain cells—from the damaging effects of free radicals.

Your brain is more vulnerable to free radical damage than just about any other part of you. In part, that's because the brain uses a lot of oxygen. It takes up just 2 percent of your body but uses about 20 percent of the oxygen—and the more oxygen your brain cells burn, the more free radicals they create. Your brain also contains large amounts of fat. In fact, nearly 50 percent of your brain by weight is fat. The hydroxyl radical is particularly damaging to fatty tissues, which means your brain is the part of your body most likely to be damaged.

Fortunately, melatonin is especially good at protecting your brain. It's made right in the very center of your brain by your pineal gland. Once melatonin is produced, it can easily slip through the blood-brain barrier that screens out a lot of other substances. It thus enters your brain cells—and their delicate membranes and mitochondria—and shields them from oxidative damage. That, in turn, may well protect you from Alzheimer's disease, memory problems, and other degenerative brain diseases, such as Parkinson's disease.

This brain protection works in two ways. First, melatonin acts as a direct free radical scavenger. According to the leading researcher in the field, Russel J. Reiter, melatonin mops up hydroxyl and peroxyl radicals "more efficiently than other known antioxidants."[6] In fact, melatonin is easily ten times as efficient as glutathione for neutralizing free radicals.[7]

It also has a stimulating effect on your antioxidant enzymes. Recent research shows that it boosts your production of SOD and glutathione. Easily entering lipids—and thus the membranes of your cells—the melatonin helps stabilize the cells and make them more resistant to oxidative attack.[8] At the same time, it slides into the mitochondria within the cells and becomes the ideal antioxidant nutrient.

These are just some of the most recent breakthroughs in melatonin research. The literature to date comprises nearly 6,000 scientific articles on the subject. Even the august *New England Journal of Medicine* conceded in a

1997 article that melatonin had significant antioxidant abilities, could strengthen the immune system, inhibited some tumors, and probably induced sleep.[9]

Just as important, melatonin has been shown to be extremely safe. Doses of up to 6 grams have no toxic effects, although they will make you sleepy or slow your reaction time. In a recent clinical trial, 1,400 women in the Netherlands took 75 mg a day for up to four years with no ill effects.

We're therefore talking about a safe, inexpensive, easily available supplement that provides outstanding antioxidant and antiaging protection. But, since it's a hormone, the only way to raise your melatonin level is to take supplements. I recommend to all my patients over the age of fifty a starting dose of 0.3 mg; over time, doses of up to 5 mg are quite safe.

To avoid any problems from the sleepiness melatonin can cause, take the dose about half an hour before bedtime. As a bonus, you'll get a more refreshing night's sleep, and as you'll learn in Chapter 13, that can do more for you than you may know.

There are, however, a few cautions for melatonin. Pregnant women should avoid it. So should women who are trying to get pregnant, because in high doses melatonin acts as a contraceptive. Because melatonin stimulates the immune system, people with autoimmune diseases or severe allergies shouldn't take it. For the same reason, people with such immune system cancers as lymphoma or leukemia should stay away from melatonin.

So far I've been discussing ways to raise your antioxidant levels through the use of vitanutrient supplements. The second prong of my approach to boosting your antioxidant levels is through a diet rich in nutrient-dense, high-antioxidant, low-carbohydrate foods. There are so many of these foods that I'll have to spend the next two chapters discussing them.

10

Ever wonder why blueberries are blue or tomatoes are red? It's because plants, like people, need free radical protection and have evolved special substances called phytochemicals to do the job. These phytochemicals—literally, plant chemicals, from the Greek *phytos*, for "plant"—give the plants their characteristic colors and flavors. Miraculously—if also logically—the phytochemicals provide similar protection to the people who eat the plants. Even more miraculously, the most colorful and protective plants are also the tastiest. As you'll discover in this chapter, vegetables and fruits are crammed with antioxidants and other substances that make all the difference to your health. If your diet is high in fresh vegetables and fruits, it's high in all kinds of protective vitanutrients. In addition, we can use supplements containing concentrated phytochemicals to help treat and prevent specific health problems.

The evidence in favor of phytochemicals from a diet rich in fruits and vegetables is overwhelming. Hundreds of recent studies show that the antioxidants in fruits and vegetables slow brain aging, reduce your risk of just about every kind of cancer, protect your eyesight, and help prevent heart disease. Antioxidant phytochemicals also prevent diabetes and help reduce diabetic complications.

Researchers have already identified thousands of phytochemicals, and there are probably thousands more waiting to be discovered. So it is very good news that this very promising area is justifiably the focus of considerable research attention. I look forward to the day when we understand the phytochemicals and what they do so precisely that doctors will prescribe foods instead of pharmaceuticals to treat and prevent most illnesses. Though it may not be in my lifetime, I firmly believe that in this century we will look back at the twentieth century's dependence on drugs instead of diet in the same way we now look back at the nineteenth century's dependence on leeches and bloodletting—as crude, ineffective, and even harmful treatments based on ignorance.

We're going to explore the two major categories of phytochemicals—carotenoids in this chapter, bioflavonoids in the next.

CAROTENOIDS

One of the most important clans within the phytochemical family, the carotenoids are a group of yellow-, orange-, and red-colored substances found in a wide variety of foods. As the name suggests, it's the carotenoids, especially one called beta-carotene, that give carrots their orange color. Carotenoids offer similar tints to squash and tomatoes, but many high-carotenoid foods, like kale, are actually dark green. The carotenoids are still in there, they're just covered up by the green phytochemicals in the plant.

The carotenoid clan is enormous. So far, researchers

have identified more than seven hundred different carotenoids, of which as many as fifty might be absorbed and used by the human body. We still don't know what, if anything, most of the carotenoids do for you if you eat them, because only fourteen or so have ever been found in human serum.[1] The relative handful of carotenoids that have been carefully studied, however, show that these phytochemicals provide powerhouse protection against free radical damage.

Some very interesting recent research also correlates carotenoids with protection from diabetes. Researchers at the federal Centers for Disease Control and Prevention looked at the levels of six major carotenoids—alpha-carotene, beta-carotene, cryptoxanthin, lutein, zeaxanthin, and lycopene—in more than one thousand people age forty to seventy-four with normal glucose tolerance. They then compared those levels to the levels of the carotenoids in 277 people with impaired glucose tolerance and in 148 people with newly diagnosed diabetes. Are you surprised to learn that the beta-carotene and lycopene concentrations were highest in the people with normal glucose tolerance, lower in those with impaired glucose tolerance, and lowest of all in the people with diabetes? I wasn't. This is yet another reason not to allow your sugar tolerance to become impaired.[2]

Let's look more closely at the carotenoids.

The Carotenes

In previous chapters, I've talked at length about the antioxidant vitamins, especially vitamins C and E. You may have wondered why I left out vitamin A. It's true that vitamin A is a valuable antioxidant. It's also true that one of vitamin A's main jobs in your body is preventing infection, so I often recommend vitamin A supplements as part of the treatment for infections and wounds, lung disease, and other serious health problems. For basically healthy people, however, there's a better way to get all the vitamin A you need and also get extra antioxidant protection: consume carotenes. Here's why.

While some of the vitamin A you get from your diet comes from egg yolks, milk, and liver, most comes from plant foods that contain alpha- and beta-carotene, which your body easily converts into vitamin A in your small intestine and liver. (Foods also contain gamma-carotene, but it doesn't seem to do much.) Only about 20 percent of the alpha-carotene you eat gets turned into vitamin A. The rest circulates in your system and enters your fatty tissues, where it is particularly good at mopping up the singlet oxygen radical and preventing lipid peroxidation, that is, damage to the fatty cell membranes.[3] There isn't that much alpha-carotene in foods compared to the amount of beta-carotene, but your body absorbs more of it from foods.

Beta-carotene is much more abundant and much more active than the alpha, by which I mean your body converts it into vitamin A very easily. But only about 40 percent of the beta-carotene that you eat turns into vitamin A. What happens to the rest? Like alpha-carotene, it circulates in your body and enters fatty tissues, where it acts as a very powerful antioxidant that protects you against heart disease and cancer. As a bonus, beta-carotene is also a major immune system booster.

For optimal absorption and use of high-carotene foods, you need to eat them with some dietary fat. If you're on a low-fat diet, you won't absorb your carotenes particularly well. And here's another important point about the carotenes: They're carried around your system by your LDL cholesterol.[4] Yes, you read that correctly. Aren't you amazed to learn that "bad" cholesterol does good things for you, despite the way it's been demonized by the medical establishment? This is a good example of how your cholesterol can indeed be too low: You can't get the benefit of beta-carotene if you don't have enough LDL cholesterol to transport it around your body. In a good example of how your body has been created to be in balance, beta-carotene also raises your level of HDL cholesterol![5]

You've probably read or heard a lot about beta-carotene in the last few years; it's become a controversial subject. I'll get to the controversy in a page or two, but first, let's set down what is known to be true about this valuable vitanutrient.

In general, people whose diets are rich in beta-carotene have lower risk of heart disease. An ongoing study of older Dutch adults showed exactly how much less. The study looked at the eating habits of nearly five thousand healthy men and women between the ages of fifty-five and ninety-five for four years. At the start of the study, none of the people had ever had a myocardial infarction (heart attack). At the end of the study, the people whose diets were highest in beta-carotene had a 45 percent reduction in their risk of a myocardial infarction compared to those whose diets were lowest in beta-carotene. The protective effect of the beta-carotene was even higher among the smokers in the group; their risk of a heart attack was cut by 55 percent. Among former smokers, the risk dropped by 68 percent.[6]

Beta-carotene is one of the safest of all vitanutrients. It would be very difficult to overdose on it, even at more than 150 mg a day for months. At worst, your skin may turn a harmless orange color (the color fades away if you cut back your dose).[7] For patients with heart disease, the beta-carotene dose I would usually prescribe is 50 mg a day.

Why does beta-carotene work so well against heart

disease? As do other antioxidants such as vitamin C and vitamin E, beta-carotene keeps LDL cholesterol from oxidizing. Remember, the only scientifically supported part of the cholesterol legend is the harm wrought when LDL cholesterol gets oxidized.

Despite the evidence in favor of beta-carotene, many conventional doctors don't recommend it for their patients. If they have any reasons beyond a reflex negative attitude toward vitanutrients, they usually mention the results of the long-term Physicians' Health Study, which failed to show any benefit of beta-carotene in reducing the risk of heart disease or cancer.[8] (Or did it? I'll get to that a little later.)

Besides the fact that the beta-carotene used in the Physicians' Health Study was synthetic and contained no other carotenoids, there was another big problem with it: The doctors involved took only 50 mg every other day. Even though they took the supplements faithfully over twelve years, 25 mg a day is just barely enough to have any positive effect. Many researchers believe the optimal amount for cancer prevention is at least 40 mg a day. As a basis of comparison, the average American takes in only about 2 mg a day from food. The above-average American who actually eats a lot of fresh vegetables gets no more than 10 mg or so from his or her daily diet. Getting 40 mg a day from food is *very* difficult—you'd have to eat about four cups of cooked carrots. The best way to be sure you're getting beta-carotene protection is through supplements.

If beta-carotene is solid protection against heart disease, it is also effective in the fight against cancer—for both prevention and treatment. But here's where this valuable vitanutrient becomes controversial, so let's deal with the controversy first.

In 1996, the Beta Carotene and Retinol Efficacy Trial

study, better known as the CARET study, showed that taking beta-carotene supplements actually increased the rates of lung cancer in smokers.[9] The medical establishment seized on this study as a way to discredit the whole idea of vitanutrients. As a result, a lot of people got the mistaken idea that beta-carotene causes all sorts of cancer in everyone.

Not so. The people in the study were all smokers, former smokers, or asbestos workers—people who were already at very high risk for lung cancer. Only the asbestos workers and the people who continued to smoke had an increased risk of lung cancer; the former smokers had a slightly reduced risk. Many of the smokers also drank alcohol, and we know that smoking and drinking severely reduce the amount of beta-carotene in your blood. Finally, the study participants took synthetic, not natural, beta-carotene supplements.

Several hypotheses have been offered to explain why the beta-carotene supplements triggered lung cancer in some of the study participants. Since we know that taking large doses of beta-carotene may keep you from absorbing other carotenes, one possibility is that the beta-carotene supplements reduced the participants' absorption of other equally valuable carotenes, such as lutein, from their food. Another is that the beta-carotene supplements may actually increase free radical production. How? By increasing your beta-carotene levels, and not simultaneously increasing your vitamin E and vitamin C levels, the cascade of chemical reactions that neutralizes free radicals gets out of balance, allowing the radicals to get the upper hand.[10] Another study in animals suggests a different hypothesis: that beta-carotene supplements increase the production of cell enzymes that interact with the carcinogenic substances in cigarette smoke, causing cancer.[11]

We do know, however, from a number of other positive studies, that among nonsmokers, beta-carotene truly does have a positive effect on the lungs, protecting them not only against cancer but also against chronic pulmonary obstructive disease, including asthma, bronchitis, and emphysema. In fact, according to a recent study of more than 18,000 adults, the more antioxidant vitanutrients such as vitamin C, vitamin E, selenium, and beta-carotene in your diet, the better your lung function is likely to be. The differences between the nonsmokers with the highest blood antioxidant levels and those with the lowest were dramatic—roughly equivalent to the difference between a nonsmoker and someone who smoked a pack a day for ten years.[12] The study also showed, however, that beta-carotene has little or no positive effect on smokers.

What conclusions can we draw from all this? First, if you smoke, stop. Second, if my words, for some strange reason, don't result in your automatically quitting, then at least start eating high-antioxidant foods and supplement your diet with full-spectrum natural carotenoids, rather than with synthetic beta-carotene.

Smoker or not, eating foods rich in carotenoids—as opposed to taking supplements—could do a lot to protect you against cancer of all sorts, including lung cancer.[13] As with heart disease, people who eat a lot of foods rich in beta-carotene, such as spinach, kale, and squash, have a reduced risk of cancer. I don't begin to have room to discuss every study that shows how effective dietary beta-carotene is for cancer prevention, but almost all of them are attributed to full-spectrum carotenoids being taken as food. To look at just one excellent recent example, a Swedish study of postmenopausal women showed that a diet rich in beta-carotene appears to lower the risk of breast cancer. And the longer the women had been eating a high-beta-carotene diet, the better protected they were.[14]

When it comes to prostate cancer, however, supplements of beta-carotene may make a big difference. Remember the Physicians' Health Study that supposedly showed no cancer prevention benefit from beta-carotene? Researchers have been looking at the results a little more closely recently, and they're starting to backpedal. Among the 22,000 male doctors taking part in the study, half were assigned to take beta-carotene supplements in addition to their normal diets. Overall, the doctors who didn't eat many fruits and vegetables had low blood levels of beta-carotene and were one-third more likely to develop prostate cancer. The men who took the beta-carotene supplements, however, were 36 percent less likely to develop prostate cancer, even if they skipped their fruits and vegetables. In this instance, the beta-carotene supplements seem to have made up for the lack of dietary carotenoids.[15]

The antioxidant power of beta-carotene is one way it fights cancer. Another reason that beta-carotene helps cancer patients is that it keeps their cells communicating properly with each other. Many carcinogens disrupt cell-to-cell communications. That lets the cancer cells get a foothold before your immune system realizes it and has a chance to react. Beta-carotene helps keep open those lines of communication—technically, the gap junctions. Even after cancer has started, restoring gap junction communication with extra beta-carotene may help reverse the process.[16]

My first mentor in the treatment of cancer was the late Dr. Hans Nieper of Hannover, Germany. Dr. Nieper was world-famous for the number of cancer survivors he had treated. A mainstay of his therapy was beta-carotene, always given in doses high enough to produce a harmless yellowing of the palms of his patients. Nieper taught me that beta-carotene helps activate the thymus gland, one of your body's most important sources of immune protection. Beta-carotene also inactivates our own suppressor cells, the lymphocytes that turn off our immune responses.[17] Dr. Nieper's brilliant work was confirmed for me yet again when I read that researchers recently showed that beta-carotene also stimulates the activity of your natural killer cells. These are the immune cells that destroy cancerous cells and that are considered by researchers to be the white blood cells most involved in fighting cancer.[18]

For patients with active cancer, I generally prescribe at least 75,000 IU of beta-carotene daily. I use natural beta-carotene extracted from a type of alga called *Dunaliella salina*. Dr. Nieper used a dry powder with special electrical charges. This may also explain the discrepancy between Nieper's success and the failures of synthetic beta-carotene.

Overall, beta-carotene is an excellent way to stimulate your immune system to fight off viruses and infections.[19] In fact, I often prescribe beta-carotene for my patients with chronic viral infections. Some of the beta-carotene is converted to vitamin A, which enhances immunity, but the beta-carotene also seems to help independent of its vitamin A activity.

Lycopene

Of all the carotenoids, lycopene is the one that's most effective for neutralizing the damaging singlet oxygen free radical.[20] Lycopene is the phytochemical that makes tomatoes red. Small amounts of lycopene are also found in watermelon and pink grapefruit, but for dietary lycopene, tomatoes are pretty much the only choice. And as we'll see in a moment, tomato juice and puree are the best ways to consume them.

All the recent research suggests that some of the benefits we once attributed to beta-carotene actually come from lycopene. In fact, lycopene offers more cancer protection than beta-carotene, perhaps as much as ten times more. It also offers more protection against LDL cholesterol oxidation, so lycopene is very good for protecting your arteries and heart against plaque formation.

You probably first began hearing about lycopene back in 1995, when reports that it helps prevent prostate cancer first came out. That first study showed that men who eat at least ten servings a week of tomato-based foods are up to 45 percent less likely to develop prostate cancer.[21] And among men who do develop prostate cancer, treatment with lycopene may decrease tumor size and make the cancer less aggressive.[22]

Interestingly, the original study showed that the most common source of lycopene for the men who ate a lot of it was tomato sauce. Like beta-carotene, lycopene can be absorbed into your body only if you eat it with some dietary fat. It's also best absorbed if it has been heated to release the lycopene from within the tomato cells, so your best dietary sources are tomato sauce and tomato paste made with olive oil. (For more information about exactly how much lycopene can be found in tomatoes and other foods, see Chapter 21.)

Since that first announcement, lycopene has been shown to help prevent other cancers as well, including cancers of the lung, stomach, colon, and breast. In fact, eating a lot of lycopene seems to reduce your overall risk of cancer by about 40 percent.[23] Smokers with low lycopene levels, for example, have four times more lung cancer than those with the highest levels.[24]

In addition to its potent antioxidant power, lycopene helps prevent tumor formation by slowing or even blocking DNA synthesis within cancer cells. That keeps the cells from reproducing. Lycopene also seems to block insulinlike growth factor 1, a hormone you make naturally that cancer cells can easily hijack and use to fuel their own growth. Stop the cancer cells with lycopene, and you slow tumor growth.

Lycopene's value isn't limited to cancer. A major study of European men compared the lycopene levels in men who had just had a first heart attack to those in healthy men. The ones who had the highest lycopene levels were half as likely to have a heart attack as those with the lowest levels.[25]

The latest research on lycopene suggests that it may also have a positive effect on your immune system. In a small study involving ten women, the ones who ate tomato puree every day for twenty-one days had higher blood levels of lycopene than the women who ate a tomato-free diet. The white blood cells of the tomato-eaters were much more resistant to oxidative damage, by anywhere from 33 to 42 percent more.[26] Even though this study was small, it is important because it ties in the improvements in lycopene levels to something of known clinical significance for strengthening your immune system.

From my perspective, the problem with dietary lycopene is that it's valuable only if it's been processed. That's not bad in itself. The real problem is finding a way to eat two servings a day of tomato sauce or tomato paste that doesn't also involve a lot of carbohydrates like spaghetti. Those who need a major reduction in their carbohydrates should take a look at Table 21.4, which lists the carbohydrate-to-lycopene ratio of various foods. Select the foods that give you the best ratio, such as tomato puree or tomato juice. Even these foods tend to be high in carbohydrates, which is why many of my patients prefer to take lycopene in supplement form.

Lutein and Zeaxanthin

Among people over fifty, the leading cause of blindness is age-related macular degeneration (AMD), or loss of central vision. About 13 million Americans have AMD, and nearly 25 percent of people over sixty-five have at least early signs of it. About 300,000 people go blind from AMD every year.

Sadly, well over half of all AMD cases could be avoided through two simple steps: stop smoking and eat foods high in the carotenes lutein and zeaxanthin. Smokers are two and a half times as likely to develop AMD as nonsmokers.[27]

Because your eyes are exposed to sunlight all the time, their tissues need to be very high in antioxidants to prevent damage caused by blue and ultraviolet light. Lutein and zeaxanthin are yellow—they give corn its color. These two carotenes are concentrated in your macula, the most sensitive area of the light-gathering retina at the back of your eye. Logic suggests they must be there for a purpose. Of course they are. They form a yellowish deposit there that absorbs blue light, which keeps it from generating damaging free radicals.

I could make a strong case for calling macular degeneration a vitamin deficiency disease, just like scurvy.[28] The only difference is that macular degeneration takes decades to show up. The best way to protect your eyes is by eating a diet rich in lutein and zeaxanthin. For lutein, that means mostly the dark-green leafy vegetables like kale and spinach. For zeaxanthin, it means the yellow foods like corn and orange peppers. Zeaxanthin is less abundant in food than lutein, but fortunately, your body also converts some lutein into zeaxanthin. The more the better: According to a recent study, people who ate the most foods rich in lutein and zeaxanthin had a 43 percent lower risk of developing AMD than those who ate the lowest amounts of these foods.[29]

What often gets left out of discussions of dietary ways to prevent AMD is the fact that egg yolks are the very best source of lutein and zeaxanthin. In fact, egg yolks contain higher concentrations of these carotenes than any other food.[30] Can't you just imagine how much macular degeneration could have been prevented if egg yolks hadn't been seen as a dietary enemy for so long? Now you know how repulsed I am every time I see a hotel breakfast menu indicating that an egg-white omelet is a "healthy" choice, which you can get for an extra fifty cents. Next time you see that, think of me, think of your eyesight, and order a spinach omelet. See if you can get the waiter to throw in some leftover egg yolks from the AHA-victimized egg-white devotees.

Macular degeneration can't be cured, but it can be slowed and even reversed a bit with vitanutrients. In one experiment, 102 people with macular degeneration took daily antioxidant vitanutrients, including vitamin C, vitamin E, beta-carotene, and selenium. In 60 percent of the cases, deterioration of the macula stopped or improved.[31] If the program had included lutein and zeaxanthin supplements, I believe it would have worked for more of the patients. At the Atkins Center, we use such a combination of vitanutrients to treat AMD. The primary carotenoid supplement is 6 to 10 mg of lutein daily. Our ace-in-the-hole for AMD is the amino acid 1-taurine, which we prefer to give intravenously.

THE ATKINS RX FOR CAROTENE SUPPLEMENTS

Since the research is still unclear as to whether taking beta-carotene supplements alone could trigger cancer in some people, I much prefer to have my patients take natural mixed-carotene supplements. These supplements contain all the carotenes, not just beta-carotene, so you get the complete antioxidant protection package. For basically healthy people, I suggest at least 10,000 IU daily, and preferably more—up to 25,000 IU. Supplements made from an algae called *Dunaliella salina* or from whole-food concentrates—provide the best mix of all the carotenes. And if you find a product that also brings in lutein, zeaxanthin, and lycopene, so much the better.

Of course, the food-processing industry, in its ingenious way, has now devised a way to completely counteract the use of carotenoids. It has created olestra, an artificial, zero-calorie fat substitute also known as Olean. Our fat-phobic society has embraced olestra, and snack foods containing the stuff are now found on supermarket shelves everywhere. Amazingly, the FDA actually approved its use, although it did insist that Procter & Gamble, the manufacturers, add vitamins A, D, E, and K to it. Why add the vitamins? Olestra is a fatty substance made from sugar and vegetable oil. It passes right through you without being digested, which means it binds up these crucial fat-soluble vitamins and carries them out of your body.

What the FDA didn't seem to care about is the way olestra also removes carotenoids. According to famed Harvard epidemiologist Meir J. Stampfer, people who eat just three small olestra-based snacks a week could expect at least a 10 percent drop in their carotenoid levels. In real terms, Stampfer projected that could mean 32,000 additional deaths from cancer and heart disease each year.[32] You already know you should stay away from junk food of any sort. Don't be snookered by advertising and the medical establishment into thinking that junk food made with olestra is somehow safe to eat, or that healthy food made with it hasn't been turned into junk food. Stick to the real thing—the foods rich in carotenoids and, as the next chapter discusses, in bioflavonoids.

11

THE BENEFITS OF BIOFLAVONOIDS

Your mother told you to eat your broccoli, and of course your mother was right—but do you know why? It's true that broccoli is full of fiber, vitamins, and minerals, all of which are good for your health. Broccoli is also crammed with health-giving phytochemicals called bioflavonoids. And whether your mother knew it or not, it's the bioflavonoids in broccoli—and in many other vegetables and fruits—that help prevent and treat a range of common health problems, including the degenerative diseases associated with aging.

The cruciferous vegetables, for example—cabbage, kale, Brussels sprouts, or the dark leafy greens like Swiss chard and beet greens—can actually sharply reduce your chances of colon cancer sharply,[1] thanks to their bioflavonoid content.

What are these substances? Bioflavonoids are made up of natural chemicals with complicated names—anthocyanosides, sulforaphane, and resveratrol—that give the foods their characteristic color and taste. They come in a range of dietary forms—vegetables, fruits, even beverages—and attack a range of illnesses. This chapter takes a look at the illnesses they prevent or treat and the foods or supplements that supply them to our bodies.

GREEN TEA: ANTIOXIDANTS IN A CUP

Tea is the most widely consumed beverage in the world, after plain water. It's also the healthiest thing you can drink, perhaps including water. Throughout the world, people who drink a lot of tea are healthier overall. In part, that could be because people who drink a lot of tea don't drink a lot of other things, like sugary soft drinks or alcohol, that are certainly bad for you. More and more, however, the evidence shows that there's more to the story than that.

What exactly is in tea? Both black and green tea contain polyphenols, chemical compounds that are powerful antioxidants and also have other useful health effects. In fact, what fascinates me is that tea seems to help just about everything, from cancer to cavities.

Ounce for ounce, green tea, made from the leaves of the plant *Camellia sinensis*, contains the most antioxidant compounds and other phytochemicals of any food or beverage there is. (Black tea, the kind most Americans drink, has been processed somewhat and has fewer bioflavonoids. Even so, black tea has almost as much health-giving value as green tea.[2])

Green tea is a valuable cancer preventive. A study in Shanghai, China, where green tea is a favorite beverage, showed that regular tea drinkers had a 50 percent lower risk of esophageal cancer.[3] A number of other studies show a similar protective effect against other cancers, including cancer of the colon, breast, lung, stomach, and skin.[4] The protective effect is greatest if you don't smoke or drink alcohol. Even so, the antitumor effect of green tea could help explain a puzzling paradox: Even though many Japanese smoke cigarettes, the lung cancer rate in Japan is surprisingly low. The reason could well be their high green tea consumption—the Japanese typically drink six cups a day or more.

How do the bioflavonoids in green tea help you? The main effect seems to come from a group of substances called catechins. Four catechins are found abundantly in green tea. The one called epigallocatechin-3-gallate (EGCG) seems to be the most exciting of all, because it has a powerful anticancer effect without side effects.[5] The EGCG probably works by inhibiting the action of an enzyme needed for cell growth. EGCG doesn't affect healthy cells, but it shuts down the enzyme in cancerous cells. Instead of continuing to reproduce wildly, the cancer cells die.[6]

YOUR HEART BENEFITS, TOO

The antioxidant bioflavonoids in tea are also a great way to protect your heart. In fact, some of the bioflavonoids in green tea are up to twenty-five times as powerful as vitamin E and one hundred times as powerful as vitamin C in quenching free radicals.[7] With that sort of antioxidant protection, it's not surprising that people who drink one or more cups of tea a day have a 46 percent reduction in heart attack risk compared to non–tea drinkers.[8]

The protection extends to your stroke risk as well. The famous Zutphen study, which looked at the stroke risk among more than 500 Dutch men over a fifteen-year period, showed that the men who had the highest intake of bioflavonoids had the lowest risk of stroke. The main source of bioflavonoids in their diet—70 percent of the total—turned out to be black tea. The men who drank more than four cups of tea a day had a two-thirds lower risk of stroke than men who drank fewer than two to three cups a day.[9]

MORE BENEFITS OF TEA

The antioxidant power of tea isn't the only thing that helps fend off heart attacks and strokes. Tea also acts as a mild anticoagulant that keeps your platelets from clumping up and making an artery-blocking clot.

The benefits of this nearly universal drink go beyond the heart as well. I think one of the most promising areas of green tea research right now is in treating arthritis. The antioxidant power of the green tea's polyphenols blocks the pathway of the Cox-2 enzyme, which is a major cause of the inflammation and pain of arthritis. The tea's polyphenols work in very much the same way as such new, heavily advertised antiarthritis drugs as Celebrex, except that the tea doesn't have the side effects, weight gain is one,—or the high cost—of the drug.[10]

Tea also has a strong antibacterial effect. Drinking a cup of tea after a meal helps prevent cavities and gum disease because the polyphenols kill the bacteria that cause these diseases. We know from other research that there's a high correlation between gum disease and heart disease. Could that be one reason for the lower heart risk among tea drinkers?

In the test tube, green tea also fights one of today's major medical problems: antibiotic-resistant bacteria. Because of thoughtless, pointless overprescribing of unnecessary antibiotics by some conventional doctors, we face today the very serious problem of dangerous bacteria that can resist the drugs we've developed to fight them. These bacteria can cause severe, even fatal infections, and they simply don't respond to drug treatment. Recent research shows that extracts of green tea may actually reverse penicillin resistance in some strains of drug-resistant bacteria. In fact, the tea seems to act synergistically with the antibiotics to make them even more potent.[11]

Of course, this work is still in the experimental stage, but I find it quite interesting. I very rarely prescribe antibiotics for my patients. Unfortunately, there are some illnesses, such as Lyme disease and the new mycoplasma epidemic, that can't really be treated with vitanutrients and diet alone. For those unusual times when I do have to prescribe antibiotics, I always want to accompany them with restoration doses of beneficial bacteria and natural substances that inhibit the growth of antibiotics' number-one complication: yeast overgrowth.

How much green tea is enough to prevent health problems is a good question. The amount of polyphenols and other bioflavonoids in a cup of freshly made tea can vary enormously. Depending on the variety of tea used and the way it was processed and brewed, there can be anywhere from 50 to 400 mg of polyphenols in a single cup. Some studies suggest that you need to sip at least six cups a day. Although, in the Shanghai study of esophageal cancer, the positive effect of green tea was noted even in people who drank only a cup a day.

I enjoy sipping a cup of tea, green or black, but to make sure my patients get the same amount of the polyphenols every time, I recommend supplements of green tea extract. Choose a brand that's standardized to contain 35 percent EGCG. If you want to avoid the caffeine in tea, look for a decaffeinated brand.

QUERCETIN

Quercetin is one of my favorite bioflavonoids, and there has been considerable research that confirms its premier status. At the Atkins Center, we use it as a major component of our allergy treatment, because quercetin naturally blocks some of the histamines your body produces in response to pollen and other allergens. The same blocking effect also works to make quercetin effective for treating inflammation of any sort, including arthritis. Quercetin is also of significant help in treating heart disease and cancer.

Like most of the bioflavonoids, quercetin acts as an anticoagulant that keeps your blood from clotting. It also protects LDL cholesterol from oxidation, which in turn prevents plaque buildup. Both effects, of course, help lower your risk of a heart attack or stroke.

Quercetin is considered the single most powerful antioxidant bioflavonoid. A new bioflavonoid called DHQ (dehydroquercetin), which may outstrip quercetin fourfold, is the one we're studying at the Atkins Center. Both are especially helpful for scavenging the peroxyl radical and preventing lipid peroxidation, the oxidative damage to such fatty parts of the body as cell membranes.[12]

As a cancer treatment and preventive, quercetin shows a lot of promise. In humans, quercetin is a valuable treatment for leukemia and breast cancer. It may well be valuable for other cancers, including colon cancer and ovarian cancer, but so far, the studies have been performed only on animals.

The best dietary source of quercetin is the humble onion. Eating one big onion, raw or cooked, is enough to raise your quercetin level noticeably within a few hours. Apples also contain quercetin, but your body can't absorb it as well; while you absorb about half the quercetin in an onion, you absorb only about 30 percent of the quercetin in an apple. Other dietary sources include tomatoes and broccoli; there's even some quercetin in green tea.

The amount of quercetin you need to help prevent disease, however, is fairly substantial. To get enough to really make a difference, you'll almost certainly need to take supplements. I usually recommend anywhere from 300 to 600 mg a day as a basic preventive against heart disease and cancer. In the case of DHQ, the equivalent dose is 200 to 500 mg daily.

Citrus bioflavonoids such as rutin, naringin, and hesperidin are closely related to quercetin. For that reason, I use the citrus bioflavonoids as part of my treatment for patients with hay fever and other allergies. For other uses, however, citrus bioflavonoid supplements aren't that effective—I prefer to use quercetin. If you want to try the citrus bioflavonoids, however, I suggest taking mixed bioflavonoids from a reliable manufacturer that specifies the amounts of each substance in the supplement.

A word of caution here: Naringinen, a citrus bioflavonoid found in grapefruit juice, can interact badly with certain drugs, particularly beta-blockers used to treat high blood pressure and angina. If you are still taking drugs such as felodipine (Plendil) or nifedipine (Procardia), don't drink grapefruit juice or take citrus bioflavonoids.*

*For information on nutritional alternatives to taking beta-blocker drugs, see *Dr. Atkins' Vita-Nutrient Solution*.

GARLIC

Pungent foods like onions and garlic are strong-tasting because they're full of valuable bioflavonoids. Garlic is so crammed with complex bioflavonoids, vitamins, and such minerals as selenium and zinc, that it's very hard to say specifically which substance gives it the most antioxidant power. The overall effect, however, is awesome: Garlic lowers your cholesterol, your triglycerides, and your blood pressure; acts as a natural anticoagulant in your blood; and is an excellent way to reduce your risk of heart disease.

In fact, garlic is so valuable that I was tempted to write a whole chapter just on its benefits. I have too many other things to say in this book, so I'll have to focus here just on garlic's antioxidant power.

Garlic has been shown in a number of studies to reduce LDL oxidation and prevent arteriosclerosis. In fact, in Germany, garlic supplements are routinely prescribed to treat arteriosclerosis. They work extremely well. A recent study in Germany showed that taking garlic supplements increases the flexibility of the aorta, the main artery carrying blood from your heart to the rest of your body. The aorta naturally stiffens with age, but the aorta of the garlic-takers in the German study was on average 15 percent more elastic than that of other men in the same age group.[13] Another German study suggests that garlic not only prevents the buildup of plaque in arteries but may even reduce it. Patients who took garlic supplements markedly slowed their rate of plaque buildup compared to the control group.[14]

Many, many laboratory experiments in the test tube and with animals show that garlic is a potent inhibitor of cancer. We don't have anywhere near as much evidence that it works in people, but I feel confident that the proof will soon be found. The research is extremely promising. For example, a compound found in aged garlic has been shown to dramatically diminish the growth of human prostate cancer cells, at least in the lab. A sulfur compound that forms as garlic ages seems to be the active ingredient.[15]

Is fresh garlic better than aged garlic extract? I like it in food, but there are advantages in using the extract, particularly for its anticancer benefits. The more garlic you take, the more benefit you get. For some people, it's easier to swallow odorless, tasteless garlic capsules than it is to eat that much garlic. I suggest a daily dose of 1,000 mg.

OPCs: POWERFUL ANTIOXIDANTS

Here's another example of valuable bioflavonoids found in foods, but in such low concentrations that you need to take supplements to get their full benefit. The oligomeric proanthocyanidins (OPCs for short) are a group of bioflavonoids found in grape seeds, berries, and the bark of some pine tree species. No matter where they come from, OPCs are powerful antioxidants, as much as fifty times more potent than equivalent amounts of vitamins C and E. They're extremely good at scavenging hydroxyl free radicals and preventing lipid peroxidation.

I find OPCs most useful for improving circulation. They carry out the particularly crucial task of building up the integrity of blood vessel walls. It's a crucial task because you need strong capillaries (the tiny blood vessels that are networked throughout your body to carry blood to all your cells). Good capillary circulation is especially important for the health of your brain, eyes, hands, and feet. OPCs restore and maintain good circulation and also reduce easy bruising, varicose veins, and other circulatory problems. They're also helpful for treating such eye problems as macular degeneration and diabetic retinopathy.

One popular way to get your OPCs is through extracts made from pine tree bark. A patented version of pine bark extract called Pycnogenol is widely sold as a dietary supplement. The OPC concentration in Pycnogenol is about 85 percent. For a slightly higher concentration of OPCs—up to 95 percent—try supplements made from grape seeds. These have the advantage of being less expensive as well. In general, I recommend taking a daily dose of 100 to 200 mg.

Anthocyanocides, the OPCs found in blueberries, bilberries (a very close Scandinavian cousin of blueberries), blackberries, red cherries, and strawberries, are also good antioxidants. Bilberries contain by far the highest concentration of anthocyanocides, which is why they're used in supplements to the exclusion of all the other berries. Bilberry supplements are very helpful for protecting your vision, especially your night vision, as you age. If you've noticed that driving at night is getting more difficult, taking bilberry supplements might help. Bilberry has also been shown to be an effective treatment for macular degeneration and diabetic retinopathy.

WHAT ABOUT WINE?

People who drink two to three glasses of red wine a day have less heart disease and cancer and live longer than nondrinkers. Recent research suggests that it's an OPC called resveratrol in the wine, not the alcohol, that does the trick.

Resveratrol is found in grape skins, so you get some whenever you drink grape juice, whether or not it's fermented. Relatively speaking, resveratrol isn't that potent an antioxidant—it's only about half as effective as OPCs. If you already habitually drink a glass or two of wine each day, you're getting some extra antioxidant protection—there's no reason to stop. If you don't usually have wine, though, there's no need to start drinking it. In fact, if you have any sort of blood sugar problem, it's best to avoid alcohol in any form. You can take resveratrol supplements, but you'll get the same benefit from grape seed supplements.

GINKGO BILOBA

Ginkgo biloba, an extract made from the leaves of the ginkgo tree, has become the latest fad supplement for inhibiting brain aging—and for good reasons, as I'll be discussing in much more detail in Chapter 18.

What's important to note here is that the antioxidant flavones that make ginkgo work so well in your brain also help other aspects of your health. I believe it's one of the most important of all the plant-based medicines. I'm hardly alone in this. In Europe, where ginkgo has been a part of standard medicine for years, it makes up nearly 1 percent of all pharmaceutical purchases. Total annual sales of ginkgo products worldwide are now over $1 billion.

More than three hundred studies demonstrate that ginkgo improves the flow of blood through your circulatory system. In fact, it's because ginkgo so greatly improves the flow of blood to your brain that it can protect your brain cells from oxidative stress and improve memory and mental function.

Elsewhere in your body, improved circulation can help treat a wide range of problems. Ginkgo supplements help improve male sexual function, stabilize irregular heart rhythms, and relieve the discomfort of intermittent claudication, a circulatory disorder in the legs. By improving circulation through the tiny blood vessels of your eyes, ginkgo also helps protect you against macular degeneration and cataracts. Similarly, improving circulation to the ears helps with such problems as hearing loss and tinnitus. Finally, ginkgo's antioxidant power is particularly effective in cleaning up the damaging superoxide radical.

Not only is ginkgo biloba extremely useful, it's also extremely safe. Even very large doses over a long period are unlikely to have any harmful effects. For patients over forty, I usually advise taking at least 60 mg three times a day. Choose a ginkgo supplement that has been standardized to contain 24 percent ginkgo bioflavonoids and 6 percent terpenes.

EAT YOUR VEGETABLES!—BUT KEEP A BALANCE

While we know what a lot of the dietary bioflavonoids do for our health, we also know that about 30 percent of the antioxidant activity of vegetables and fruits comes from bioflavonoids that haven't yet been identified. In fact, the bioflavonoids we've talked about in this chapter are merely a sample of what is known.

That's why it's important to eat a *variety* of vegetables. With variety, you get the benefit of both the known bioflavonoids and those yet to be discovered. And dietary bioflavonoids, as I've stressed over and over throughout this chapter, provide an excellent way to keep your antioxidant level high and thus protect yourself against cancer, heart disease, and all the other ailments that are supposedly a "normal" part of growing older.

Not all vegetables are created equal, however. You need to balance the total antioxidant value of a vegetable against its carbohydrate content, and some of you need to do so more than others. Sweet potatoes, for instance, are a great source of beta-carotene, minerals, and bioflavonoids, but they're also very high in carbohydrates. That means that those of you who have problems with weight, blood sugar, triglycerides, or high blood pressure might be better off looking for a different vegetable. To help you decide which vegetables give you the most bioflavonoids for the least carbohydrates, see the tables in Chapter 21.

Similarly, fruits are full of good nutrition, but they also contain a lot of fructose and glucose. Here, too, you need to balance antioxidants against carbohydrates—and simple sugars, at that. As you'll learn from the tables in Chapter 21, most fruits—with the exception of berries— are far too high in sugar for the bioflavonoids you get from them.

Learning how to achieve that balance of carbohydrate/bioflavonoid content is such a central part of your age-defying diet that all of Chapter 21 is devoted to discussing it.

We know now why we age, and we've explored some of what's available to us to counter the effects of the aging process. How can we use what we've learned? What steps can we take to slow or even reverse the aging process? In the following chapters, we go into action.

12

REVERSING DECLINING HORMONE LEVELS

You've probably noticed the impressive proliferation of "antiaging" clinics throughout the United States. A quick glance at their advertisements and brochures tells you that hormones are one of the mainstays of their treatment programs. The clinics promise to restore your hormones to the levels of your youth, when you were in the prime of life. Makes sense, you probably thought, but it sounds too good to be true.

I agree with you. It does make sense, and in fact the logic behind hormone restoration is supported by reams of scientific data. If done properly, hormone optimization or hormone rebalancing—terms I prefer over "hormone restoration"—is one of the powerful tools of age-defying medicine.

When it comes to the "too good to be true" part, that simply depends on whether the rebalancing is done properly. Doing it properly involves a thorough understanding of the interrelationships among all the hormones and an evidence-based system for knowing whether your hormonal levels—and I'm talking about all of them—are, in fact, at their individual optimal points.

In this chapter, I'll discuss the role of hormones in your body and how they can be used to help you defy the effects of aging. I'll try to simplify a highly complex subject as I introduce you to some of the most powerful weapons we have for restoring our youthful vigor and arming ourselves against the degenerative illnesses of old age.

WHAT HORMONES DO

Your body is an intricate, exquisitely balanced living machine, and it is hormones that keep the balance. They are powerful messenger chemicals that regulate every aspect of your body's functions, from your blood pressure to your body temperature to your sex drive. Created by your endocrine glands—including your adrenal glands, ovaries or testicles, thyroid, parathyroids, pineal gland, pituitary gland, and pancreas—hormones are sent into circulation in your bloodstream to travel throughout the body.

From birth until old age, much of what distinguishes you from everyone else is the relative preponderance of one hormone over another. But as we age, we all experience declines in virtually every hormone, with some declining faster than others. You already know from Chapter 5, for instance, that your resistance to the hormone insulin rises as you get older, especially in Western cultures. Your production of the hormone melatonin, made in your pineal gland, steadily declines with age. Your levels of steroid hormones—the hormones produced primarily in your adrenal and reproductive glands—drop quite rapidly as you age, so you produce less of the master hormones DHEA and pregnenolone and less of the sex hormones estrogen, progesterone, and testosterone.

With the steady drop in your hormone levels come the symptoms of aging. Your body gets weaker. You lose muscle mass and muscle tone. Your bones become brittle, your blood vessels weaken, and you are less able to resist infection. Hormone decline also affects your mind. You become less alert, more anxious, more depressed. You have trouble with short-term memory. You may have trouble sleeping soundly. Your libido declines, and you tire easily.

As your natural output of hormones inexorably declines, must your health and life span decline as well? Absolutely not. In the first place, twentieth-century scientists showed us ways to slow the decline in most of these hormones. When slowing the decline isn't enough and your body is still no longer making the hormones in sufficient quantity, we can safely replace them with hormone supplements.

HORMONE CAUTIONS

While science has shown us clearly how to use hormone supplements safely and restore our hormone levels to the peaks we experienced at age thirty, we also have the option of using hormone replacement unsafely. That's the reason—probably the only valid reason—that you're likely to read about how dangerous hormones can be.

The danger is real. Don't confuse hormone supplements with the vitamins, minerals, or other vitanutrient supplements you are taking. Although you can easily buy some hormone supplements at any health food store or pharmacy, they are potent products. Unlike most nutrients, they need to be taken in very specific doses that must be carefully measured, preferably under the supervision of an experienced physician. The goal is to achieve the ideal blood level of the hormone. Too little is inadequate. Too much can be dangerous in itself and is quite likely to throw your other hormones out of sync. So, doing it properly means not only bringing the level of an undersupplied hormone up to an optimal level, it also means keeping in balance with the other hormones.

At the Atkins Center, I use blood measurements to determine the hormone levels of my patients both before and after they start taking hormone supplements. The individual dosages are based on the starting measurements and then are adjusted up or down as needed.

I recommend the same for my readers: If you're going to reap the rewards of hormone optimization, you should find an experienced physician who can do the blood testing necessary to determine the dosages that are right for you. You also want a physician who knows the ins and outs of hormone therapy. As I'll explain a little later in this chapter, most hormones prescribed in mainstream medicine are actually unnatural variants of the hormones our endocrine glands manufacture naturally. If you take these artificial substances, you're very likely to create an imbalance within your overall hormonal profile. And hormone imbalance is something to be assiduously avoided.

Here's why. Ideally, your hormones act in concert, just as an orchestra plays together in tune. When your hormones are all working well in sync with each other, your body is working at peak harmony—the physiological equivalent of an orchestra playing a symphony, the Hormone Philharmonic in a stellar performance. But just as one instrument playing too vigorously can overpower the melodic line and throw the other musicians off, so can too much of one hormone—whether produced in your body or taken as a supplement—overpower the other hormones and suppress their action.

To avoid that, and to make sure you realize the full benefits of hormone supplementation, you need to find an experienced and expert hormone optimization specialist. It may not be all that easy; Although mainstream endocrinologists are keenly aware of the value of total hormonal balance, only a small minority of them actually take steps to help their patients achieve it. So you may have to spend some time searching out a doctor willing to work with you on this. In the future, I predict that this task will become much easier and that hormone optimization will one day be taught in medical school. In the meantime, should you find yourself seeking the help of such a specialist, I suggest you use this book as a guide to determine whether you are getting the best counseling possible.

THE HORMONE PHILHARMONIC

I've said that the most important lesson of hormone therapy is the fact that you can totally deharmonize your endocrine balance by giving it too much of a single hormone. But—and this applies mainly to the steroid hormones, the group I'll be discussing the most—some hormones are more likely to cause this problem than others. To understand which are more likely to do this, we need to look at the process of differentiation your body uses to make hormones.

It's a complex process, and it begins with that much-maligned, essential chemical building block called cholesterol. When your body determines that it needs the cholesterol more to create steroid hormones than to make bile, nerve sheaths, or any of the other cholesterol-based substances in your body, it converts the cholesterol into a rudimentary precursor chemical called a prohormone. Then, by the addition or deletion of a single molecule or a simple cluster of molecules, the prohormone is converted into a real hormone, such as an adrenal or a sex hormone.

Generally, most hormonal biochemistry proceeds easily toward differentiating into the hormones your body perceives it needs. It's biochemically almost impossible to go in the other direction and return to an earlier stage of differentiation.

Let me present, as an example, the most common hormonal abnormality I see among my patients: A woman taking a full dose of hormone replacement therapy—with unnatural estrogens and progesterones—will almost invariably have considerably depleted blood levels of DHEA, the hormone precursor I'll discuss in just a moment. This happens because of a feedback loop in which an increased level of a differentiated hormone suppresses the manufacture of an earlier form of the hormone. It means the woman is likely to be deficient in a variety of important hormones derived from DHEA.

Let's learn about this in detail.

DHEA: THE MOTHER HORMONE

DHEA, or dehydroepiandrosterone, is called "the mother hormone" because it's the precursor for the other adrenal hormones. This includes all the adrenal steroids (like the stress hormone cortisol) and all the sex hormones (like estrogen, progesterone, and testosterone). If your DHEA production drops, so does your production of all the other related hormones. It's also the most abundant hormone in your body.

But what's really special for our purposes is that, of all the biomarkers for aging, DHEA is perhaps the most telling. Study after study confirms that DHEA levels are an excellent predictor of age-related health problems:

Since our DHEA starts going down when we're in our mid-twenties, and since DHEA is probably the most rapidly declining hormone, the lower your DHEA, the more likely you are to have the degenerative diseases of accelerated aging: atherosclerosis, diabetes, cancer, osteoporosis, and lowered immunity. To put it more bluntly, the lower your DHEA, the more likely you are to die from an age-related disease.[1]

Conversely, high levels of DHEA may protect you from these same diseases—or even reverse them. And the higher your DHEA level, the better you feel, with a greater sense of overall well-being and a better ability to deal with emotional and physical stress.[2]

Your adrenal glands manufacture DHEA from cholesterol (you also make very small amounts of DHEA in your testes or ovaries). Yes, that's the same cholesterol that consensus medicine insists is a dangerous substance that has no business being in your blood, and that we keep finding essential uses for. Inadequate blood levels of cholesterol mean that your body doesn't have the essential raw materials it needs to make the crucial hormone that's the precursor for more than forty other crucial adrenal hormones. The cascade of hormone production is seriously disrupted, with predictably serious consequences for your health. Almost every patient I've given DHEA to, young or old, has shown dramatic improvement as soon as his or her DHEA level was restored to an optimal level.

After peak levels of DHEA are reached—when you're between twenty and twenty-five—the amount of DHEA you produce declines naturally at the rate of about 2 percent a year. That means that by the time you're forty or so, you're making only about half the DHEA you did at age twenty. At age sixty-five, you're down to only about 10 to 20 percent of your peak. At age eighty, you're making only about 5 percent of your peak. In general, women make about 10 to 20 percent less DHEA than men, although their rate of production still declines at the same 2 percent a year.

DHEA AND HEART DISEASE

DHEA is another excellent example of how a conventional physician's preoccupation with high cholesterol blinds him or her to other, far more decisive indicators of potential heart disease. Low DHEA is a much better predictor of a heart attack than high cholesterol, yet your doctor is very unlikely to test your DHEA level.[3] In fact, your doctor is very likely to treat your high cholesterol with a statin drug that works by preventing the manufacture of cholesterol, thereby reducing your production of DHEA even further.

Exactly the opposite approach would be far better. Taking DHEA supplements will also lower your LDL cholesterol—but without the side effects of statin drugs. At the same time, the DHEA will lower your chances of suffering a dangerous blood clot. Of course, you'll also be enjoying all the other benefits of increased DHEA levels.[4]

Animal studies suggest that if you already have atherosclerosis, DHEA might actually shrink the plaques that are clogging your coronary arteries. When rabbits with atherosclerosis are given DHEA, the plaques in their arteries shrink by 50 percent. DHEA hasn't yet been shown to reduce arterial plaque in humans, but we do know that there's a definite correlation between DHEA levels and coronary artery disease. To give just one example, a particularly interesting study of patients about to have coronary bypass operations showed that the higher their DHEA, the less severe was their coronary artery disease.[5]

ENHANCING IMMUNITY WITH DHEA

A twenty-year-old can quickly shake off a cold or flu that would keep a fifty-year-old sick for a week. As you age, your immune system grows weaker, making you more susceptible to illness, infection, and degenerative diseases like atherosclerosis and autoimmune diseases. If you could restore your immune system to its youthful level, wouldn't you?

You can, with DHEA. This amazing hormone has been shown to increase your production of antibodies and increase the activity of such infection-fighting immune cells as monocytes and natural killer cells.

In 1997, a careful study of healthy older men showed just how well DHEA enhances immunity. The test subjects took 50 mg of DHEA a day for twenty weeks. At the end of that time, all the men showed remarkable increases in immune components in their blood. Most notably, their monocytes increased on average by 45 percent, while other immune markers, such as T cells, went up by at least 20 percent.[6]

I see the evidence for the immune-enhancing function of DHEA every day in my patients. At the Atkins Center, we prescribe it for all patients with impaired immunity. It's particularly effective for patients with chronic fatigue syndrome or such autoimmune ailments as rheumatoid arthritis and lupus. Virtually all of these patients have surprisingly low levels of DHEA; after they have been on DHEA for just a few weeks, I see a strong improvement in their overall immune function.

Equally important, the patients feel much better, and symptoms of depression and fatigue are usually much improved, if not gone.

CANCER AND DHEA

It's not a cure, but DHEA could be something even better: a supplement that prevents cancer to begin with. I first learned about the use of DHEA as a therapy in the 1970s, when alternative oncologists in Germany began using it successfully with their cancer patients.

So far, most of the medical evidence on DHEA is from animal studies, but I'm optimistic that the positive outcomes will translate into similar results for humans. These animal studies show that DHEA prevents cancers of the breast, colon, liver, lungs, prostate, lymphatic system, and skin. We know that your chances of getting cancer rise as your DHEA levels fall. We also know from human studies that people with bladder cancer and women with breast cancer always have much lower than normal DHEA levels.[7] All the evidence points toward a strong role for DHEA as a cancer preventive, even if the definitive studies have yet to be done.

One known exception: A man at risk for prostate cancer, or one who already has it, needs to be very cautious about using DHEA. I believe you can still benefit from this helpful hormone, but you do need to be monitored carefully by a physician. That's because DHEA can increase your testosterone production, which in turn could feed your prostate cancer. To use DHEA safely, you need to have frequent prostate-specific antigen blood tests (PSA tests) to monitor your risk of prostate cancer. A useful alternative here is 7-keto DHEA, a variation that leads to the development of the adrenal hormones but not to the production of testosterone or other sex hormones.

STRONGER BONES WITH DHEA

DHEA not only can stop osteoporosis, it can reverse it. It does so by increasing the activity of bone-building cells called osteoblasts and inhibiting the activity of bone-destroying cells called osteoclasts.

People who have osteoporosis have much lower levels of DHEA than people who don't. Similarly, among older adults, the people with the highest DHEA levels have the densest bones. We know from animal studies that DHEA supplements can actually restore lost bone density.[8] Can it do the same for you? I think it can, which is why I use DHEA supplements to create optimal blood levels for all my patients—male and female—who are at risk for osteoporosis.

TAKING DHEA

All of these wonderful DHEA benefits strongly suggest that you should be aware of your DHEA level and supplement it if it's low. To determine your DHEA level, I prefer to do a blood test that measures your level of DHEA-S, the sulfated form of DHEA. Since about 90 percent of the DHEA in your body is in this form, the test provides a fairly accurate assessment. While most mainstream doctors assume a very broad "normal" range and correlate it to your age, I have found no problems trying to restore the DHEA blood levels of my patients to what is optimal for a thirty-year-old. In older patients, in fact, that is the goal: to achieve the level of someone in his or her twenties or thirties. For women, that's ideally between 200 and 300 units; for men, it's between 300 and 400.

THE CORTISOL CONNECTION

As a basic rule, hormonal imbalance is unlikely. It just doesn't happen very easily. The process of differentiation that develops precursor prohormones into a range of differentiated hormones is so varied, and the body offers so many differentiation options, that balance is easy to achieve, especially since the body itself determines which derivatives it needs most. If you're taking hormone supplements, and your body suddenly finds it has too much or too little of other hormones, feedback mechanisms spring into action and turn off the flow of what's in excess, or speed up production of what's needed.

But DHEA and its companion prohormones are among the few hormones in your body that don't have a feedback mechanism. Your body, so far as we know, doesn't respond to DHEA supplements by shutting down its own DHEA production.

Instead, your normal DHEA production is counteracted, in a very complex process, by the adrenal hormone cortisol. Sometimes called the stress hormone, cortisol is made in your adrenal glands and secreted when your body needs it. It's the second most abundant hormone in your body after DHEA. When you're under stress, however, you make extra cortisol, and that inhibits your production of DHEA. As time goes by and you age, the combination of naturally decreasing DHEA production plus the continual stress many of us are under from work and family pressures leads to a relative increase in cortisol, which can prove to be a serious hormonal imbalance. Your DHEA production, already naturally lower, gets further suppressed by excess cortisol. Your hormonal harmony tips out of balance as the cortisol gradually takes over. Instead of a symphony, you have cacophony.

A situation of too much cortisol and not enough DHEA has major ramifications for your health. As the cortisol pushes out the DHEA, all your other hormones are affected as well. In particular, the cortisol-DHEA connection is closely related to the insulin-glucagon connection. As your cortisol level rises, so does your insulin level. Once you start getting excess cortisol in your system, the aging process accelerates. Not only do you lose the protection of DHEA, the cortisol also inhibits your production of eicosanoids, the short-lived chemical messengers that carry out the order sent by your hormones.

Clearly, restoring the balance between your DHEA and cortisol levels is of crucial importance to breaking this deadly aging cycle. One major step in that direction is to reduce your cortisol level, so that your body will be able to make and use as much of your natural DHEA as possible. Because cortisol is the stress hormone, one good way to lower your levels of it is to lower your stress levels. There are some vitanutrients that serve well to bring those levels down, for example, acetyl-l-carnitine, vitamin C, vitamin A, zinc, and selenium.

DHEA DOSES

The other side of the DHEA-cortisol reduction equation is the dosage of your DHEA supplements. As a starting dose, I generally prescribe 10 to 30 mg of DHEA to a woman and 30 to 50 mg to a man. I use follow-up DHEA-S levels to adjust the dose until the desired blood level is reached. DHEA has very few side effects, but at high doses there may be unwanted hair growth in women, acne, irritability, and insomnia. In some very rare cases, people taking high doses may develop heart palpitations or irregular heartbeats.

Although DHEA is the precursor hormone to estrogen, in practice it doesn't seem to raise estrogen levels much if at all. Almost all of a woman's estrogen is produced in her ovaries. Based on the current research, it's unlikely that taking DHEA supplements will raise your risk of breast cancer. In fact, DHEA has long been part of the breast cancer *treatment* protocols of several European alternative cancer therapists.

Today many reputable manufacturers produce pharmaceutical-grade DHEA. To make DHEA, a sterol called diosgenin is extracted from wild yams. Diosgenin needs to be manipulated through at least six steps in the laboratory to convert it into DHEA. You may encounter products that claim to be "wild yam extract," "DHEA precursor," or "natural DHEA." Since your body can't begin to transform wild yam extract into DHEA, these products are not what you're looking for. Don't consider any product whose label doesn't clearly state the dose of DHEA in milligrams.

PREGNENOLONE: THE GRANDMOTHER HORMONE

If DHEA is the mother hormone, then pregnenolone can be called is the "grandmother" hormone. Cholesterol in your body is converted to pregnenolone as the first biochemical step in making all your other steroid hormones.

In fact, pregnenolone is the direct precursor of DHEA. The body converts it into a range of other hormones, such as androstenedione and androstenediol, which are then converted into the hormones testosterone and estradiol and its derivatives, cortisol, and aldosterone.

Pregnenolone was first discovered back in the 1940s, when researchers found that adrenal hormones could suppress the pain and swelling of rheumatoid arthritis. Pregnenolone, they discovered, was the only hormone that helped relieve the symptoms without the metabolic side effects the other hormones induced. Despite this, they turned their attention to hydrocortisone and its derivatives and eventually came up with the corticosteroid drugs, like prednisone, that were originally hailed as "miracle drugs." Today these drugs are seen for what they are: dangerous artificial substances that cause such a wide range of adverse side effects they cannot be taken in high doses for more than a brief period.

At the Atkins Center, we use natural pregnenolone supplements—generally in conjunction with DHEA—to treat problems that conventional physicians treat with prednisone. Pregnenolone isn't quite as powerful or fast-acting, but it is much less likely to raise your blood pressure, lead to weight gain, give you diabetes, or make you retain fluids. We find it to be very helpful for treating arthritis and such autoimmune diseases as lupus and multiple sclerosis. Since we feel that pregnenolone and DHEA should be in balance, we use comparable amounts of each.

Recent research indicates that pregnenolone can also help with one of the most annoying problems of aging: short-term memory loss. You've probably noticed that your short-term memory isn't what it used to be. You can't remember new names and faces as well as you used to, and you may be starting to misplace minor items like a pen or your car keys. Pregnenolone holds out the promise of being a safe and truly effective memory-enhancing drug. The work on this is still in the preliminary stages, but the most recent studies strongly suggest that pregnenolone improves memory in older adults, at least as measured by standard memory tests.[9]

Pregnenolone's main advantage, however, is that it is also converted into progesterone. Because that conversion takes place one step before pregnenolone is converted into DHEA, the grandmother hormone can serve as a vital hormone for women by creating a balance with estrogen. I'll come back to this point for more discussion in the next chapter, when I talk about turning back the clock with hormones.

Your pregnenolone production peaks when you're in your early thirties and then steadily declines. By the time you reach your seventies, your pregnenolone production is down to just about 40 percent of your peak.[10] A decline in pregnenolone production is a natural part of growing older, but you can accelerate the decline unnaturally by starving your body of cholesterol. An overly strict, cholesterol-free vegetarian diet could deprive you of the essential raw material from which pregnenolone is made. Another path to pregnenolone deprivation is provided by the statin family of cholesterol-lowering drugs. If you're on a cholesterol-free diet, or if you're taking statin drugs, you have a good shot at unnaturally reduced pregnenolone production. And since pregnenolone is the grandmother hormone, making less of it—for whatever reason—means you also make less of all the other hormones down the line, with all the predictable negative consequences.

The natural decline in pregnenolone production is seen as one reason why your DHEA production drops as you age, as does your production of the enzyme that converts pregnenolone to DHEA. Taking pregnenolone supplements, which are now available over the counter, may not increase your DHEA level. Taking pregnenolone and DHEA supplements together, however, could do a lot to restore optimal levels of both hormones. It may have the additional advantage of turning down your production of cortisol. Remember, pregnenolone is the master hormone for both the desirable DHEA and the far less desirable cortisol. Taking pregnenolone and DHEA together seems to keep the pregnenolone from being converted to cortisol.

To help restore youthful levels of pregnenolone in my patients, I usually start with doses of from 20 to 40 mg daily. If, after a few months, the level hasn't gone up enough, I might raise the dose until it does. How you will react to pregnenolone is unpredictable. Don't try taking supplements on your own. You need to work with an experienced physician who can use blood tests at regular intervals to monitor your levels and optimize your dosage.

Hormone optimization is a complex subject, and its impact—helping you regain some of your youthful vigor and health—is just the first step. In the next chapter I'll explain how you can improve your levels of hormones in such a way as truly to turn back the clock.

13

HORMONES THAT TURN BACK THE CLOCK

Can any single hormone truly turn back the clock on aging? Can any one vitanutrient bring you back to the youthful health and vigor you enjoyed in your twenties and thirties? No. There are no magic bullets against aging. But it is the entire premise of this book that the right *combination* of vitanutrients, along with the right diet and lifestyle, can certainly slow the clock, perhaps stop it, and maybe even roll it back a bit.

In the previous chapter, we looked at ways to retard or stop the decline in hormone level and thus arm yourself against the degenerative illnesses of aging. In this chapter, we'll take the use of hormones a step farther—from stopping decline to proactively enhancing your vigor. You'll learn about the vitanutrients that are most effective for restoring low levels of such steroid hormones as testosterone and progesterone. You'll also learn about natural, safe ways to eliminate menopause symptoms and lower your risk of osteoporosis. And you'll learn about one of the most exciting and controversial new developments in hormone optimization, human growth hormone: what it does, how it works, and a variety of ways to build it up in your body. The combined impact of all these techniques is the closest thing there is to the legendary and still elusive Fountain of Youth.

ANDROSTENEDIONE AND NATURAL TESTOSTERONE

You don't have to be a sports fan to have heard about Mark McGwire's record-smashing seventy home runs in the 1998 season. A bit of controversy went along with the record, because McGwire openly acknowledged his use of an over-the-counter hormone supplement called androstenedione. While perfectly legal in major league baseball, the use of androstenedione is banned by many other sports organizations. The reason? The sports officials say androstenedione is an anabolic steroid, that is, a steroid hormone that builds muscle. It's therefore an unfair intrusion of something unnatural—and potentially harmful—that violates the purpose and purity of sport.

The officials, however, are more than a little off base. Androstenedione is indeed a steroid, but it's very different from the artificial anabolic steroid drugs, such as methyltestosterone, that are rightly banned in all sports. Artificial anabolic steroids, like all artificial hormones, are unnatural substances that your body is not equipped to deal with. Instead of being cleared from your system naturally and easily through your normal metabolic pathways, as are androstenedione and other natural hormones, these drugs break down into toxic by-products that can do serious harm to your liver and may even cause cancer.

More to the point, the drug hormones are not in the normal pathway of progression and differentiation of prohormones; therefore, the body cannot convert them into hormones when it happens to need more.

Since most of us aren't professional athletes, and

since androstenedione is sold legally at any pharmacy or health food store, and since it is safe to use in reasonable doses, there's no reason not to take it—if it's right for you.

But when is it right for you? That's a good question. Generally speaking, androstenedione is said to produce a brief rise in your testosterone level that lasts for only a few hours. From the few studies that have been done, it's not at all clear that androstenedione raises your testosterone level enough to have any real impact. But my experience using it in combination with DHEA indicates that a significant level of testosterone can be achieved and, in fact, serum testosterone levels can be used to monitor androstenedione dosage.

In a recent study, a group of men took 300 mg a day of androstenedione (the control group was given placebo pills) and began a weight-lifting program. At the end of the study, the men who had taken the androstenedione showed significant declines in their HDL cholesterol levels and increases in their levels of the female hormone estrogen compared to the control group. What they did not show was any increase in muscle mass or strength compared to those taking the placebo. Evidently, the power gains were the result of the weight-lifting, not the androstenedione.[1]

I often recommend androstenedione to my patients when I feel they will benefit from testosterone, and I usually give it with DHEA. The dosage is whatever produces optimal levels of DHEA and testosterone. Why are optimized testosterone levels important as an antiaging technique? Read on.

TESTOSTERONE TALES

Some of my male patients first come to me seeking help for such vague problems as fatigue, loss of muscle strength, insomnia, and depression. Others have more specific problems, perhaps heart disease or osteoporosis. And some are having the very specific problem of erectile difficulty or loss of sexual desire. What they often all have in common is low testosterone levels. They're producing only a fraction of the free testosterone they need to remain active, vital, and healthy. Testosterone levels, like most of the steroid hormones we've been discussing, drop with advancing years. But I still like to see to it that my older patients achieve levels normal for a man in his thirties.

In testing for testosterone, most conventional doctors use a blood test that measures your total testosterone. That results will almost certainly say that your testosterone level is normal. By the misleading standards of the test, it is. But now ask your doctor to do a blood test that measures your level of *free* testosterone. Since almost all the testosterone in your body is bound to a protein called sex hormone binding globulin (SHBG), or to other proteins, only about 1 to 3 percent of your testosterone is actually free—that is, bioavailable for use in your body. That's not very much, so even a small decline in your total free testosterone could have a profound effect on your health. But you won't know about it unless you do the free testosterone test, a far better measure of your true testosterone level than total testosterone.

To a degree, making less testosterone as you age is perfectly normal. Men naturally begin to make less as they enter their fifties, just as women naturally begin to produce less of the female hormones. In fact, the process in men is in many ways so similar to that in women that it's often called male menopause or andropause.

Like menopausal women, andropausal men in their late forties and early fifties experience increases in body fat, a greater risk of cardiovascular disease and osteoporosis, depression, and forgetfulness. The major difference is that a woman can use a monthly marker—her menstrual period—to be aware of the changes in her body. Men don't have a similar marker. Even if they did, many would ignore it. What man likes to think that the hormone that defines his very maleness could possibly be diminishing?

The truth, gentlemen, is that your testosterone production does slowly decline as you age, generally for one or more reasons. The most common cause is a natural decrease in the number of your Leydig cells, the testosterone-producing cells in your testes. The fewer Leydig cells you have, the less testosterone you make, and the number of Leydig cells does decrease with age. Another common cause of decreased testosterone is an increase in SHBG, the protein that binds testosterone and makes it unavailable to your body. For reasons we don't fully understand yet, you make *more* SHBG as you age.

Other factors can reduce the *activity* of your Leydig cells. An excess of the female hormone estradiol suppresses the function of the Leydig cells. All men produce some estradiol as a normal function of producing testosterone, but ordinarily, you have a good balance between lots of testosterone and a little estradiol. As you age, though, the balance can get out of whack.

One good way to throw it out of whack is to grow a spare tire around your middle. In a complicated metabolic process, the excess abdominal fat of the spare tire makes your body convert more of your testosterone into the female hormone estradiol; the fat also stores estradiol. All that extra estradiol sends a message to the pituitary gland in your brain, the master controller of your hormone production. The pituitary, in turn, sends a message to your testes telling them to turn down their testosterone production. The result is that your testosterone level drops and your estradiol level rises, with very undesirable effects on your sexuality and health.

Of course, losing that spare tire means losing weight, a project that is laughably easy to those who know my low-carbohydrate diet, as you will once you've made a commitment to follow the program I outline in *Dr. Atkins' New Diet Revolution.*

Sometimes low testosterone is caused by following the standard medical advice to eat a low-fat diet. I find this happening a lot in my patients with cardiovascular disease. Their dread of dietary cholesterol frightens them onto low-fat diets, with the hearty approval of their conventional cardiologists, and they thus starve their bodies of the cholesterol they need to make testosterone. The paradox of these misguided efforts is that testosterone has a protective effect on the heart and actually improves blood lipid profiles.[2]

Testosterone levels can be raised using a variety of supplements other than testosterone. Supplemental DHEA, which is easily converted into testosterone, is often very valuable. And I am convinced that androstenedione enhances DHEA's testosterone-raising effect. Equally critical are the anticortisol nutrients discussed in Chapter 12. When your cortisol levels are high, your DHEA levels are low—and your testosterone level is also low because you don't have enough of the precursor. Counteract the cortisol with carnitine, zinc, pantothenic acid, and other nutrients, and your DHEA level, and thus your testosterone level, will rise.

There are still some men, however, whose testosterone level fails to return to the goal level despite all these measures. In their cases, I prescribe supplements of natural testosterone. I emphasize the *natural* part of that prescription. Over the years, pharmaceutical companies have patented a wide variety of *un*natural testosterone supplements, otherwise known as anabolic steroid drugs. If these drugs were taken orally, they'd be broken down immediately by the liver. Instead, drugs such as methyltestosterone have to be administered by injection so they'll be slowly released into your bloodstream.

Recently, some drug manufacturers have discovered that although they can't patent natural testosterone, they can still profit from it by providing easy and painless ways to administer it. And so today natural testosterone is available in skin patches, skin creams and gels, and in an under-the-tongue tablet. These new delivery systems make it easy for patients to give themselves a steady, exact dose on a daily basis.

Natural testosterone is a very effective treatment, but it needs to be used with caution. In particular, men who have a history of prostate cancer should not use it— although there's no evidence to show that taking testosterone can cause prostate cancer. To be on the safe side, I always screen patients for prostate cancer using the PSA or prostate-specific antigen blood test.

A word of warning: Since taking testosterone can cause a transient rise in your PSA level, if you're planning to have a blood test to evaluate your PSA output, stay off the testosterone for a few days before.

TESTOSTERONE FOR WOMEN

All women naturally produce small amounts of testosterone, and just as a woman's production of female hormones declines with age, so too does her production of testosterone. Testosterone is essential to managing menopause. Its lack is the major reason that many menopausal women report declining libido and less satisfaction from sex, even if they are already using female hormone replacement therapy, HRT. Because the dose needed to restore a woman's normal testosterone level is quite small, I prescribe it carefully—it's easy to give too much. Sometimes, I use DHEA and/or androstenedione, which are converted naturally into testosterone in the body. When I see a measurable rise in testosterone, I know we can achieve our goal.

PROGESTERONE: MENOPAUSE THE NATURAL WAY

There may not be a more controversial area of hormone optimization than HRT for menopause. Standard medical treatment calls for women who have stopped menstruating to be given a combination of estrogen and progesterone. These artificial hormones, which differ substantially from the hormones they are said to replace, are heavily advertised in medical journals and enthusiastically endorsed by the medical establishment. Prescribing HRT for women over fifty has become almost automatic for many physicians.

The only problem is that if a woman is already hormonally imbalanced, the combination of unnatural estrogen and progesterone can be downright dangerous to her health. The combination will make most women gain weight, especially if they have a tendency to do so and even if they are at normal weight when they start. It will certainly keep women from losing weight if they are overweight. If you already have an insulin-related disorder such as low blood sugar, diabetes, high triglycerides, or high blood pressure, HRT will make the problems worse. If you're on the borderline for an insulin-related disorder, HRT could tip you over into worse health.

Whenever I wear my other hat, that of a weight-control guru with a diet able to provide weight loss in more than 99 percent of those who follow it, I note the true magnitude of the HRT problem. It inhibits weight loss, even to the point of turning my weight-loss diet into a weight-gaining experience. In case you're wondering how often that happens, I can report that I've seen it among my patients more than 3,000 times.

Here's why. Progesterone has been a known weight-gaining hormone since 1976. That's when the famed Swedish metabolic researcher Per Bjorntorp described animal studies showing an increase in the size of fat cells along with a sevenfold increase in plasma insulin levels.[3] The problems arise from progestins, the synthetic version of progesterone. As to the estrogen component of HRT, it inhibits glucagon, the one hormone that tries to neutralize the effects of insulin. Giving estradiol to women cuts down glucagon secretion and allows the blood lipids to elevate.[4]

With so much basic research indicating that HRT has adverse effects on glucose/insulin metabolism, it's amazing how few doctors who prescribe it are aware of the problems they are causing.

Do the supposed benefits of HRT balance out the disadvantages? I don't think so. The mantra conventional doctors repeat over and over is that HRT prevents cardiovascular disease. The mantra is based on numerous epidemiological studies showing that women who take hormones do considerably better in avoiding heart disease than those who do not. But a recent study, more scientifically rigorous and involving twenty medical centers nationwide, has shown that a new mantra is badly needed. Nearly three thousand women participated in the four-year Heart and Estrogen/Progestin Replacement Study (HERS), with half taking a synthetic hormone replacement formula and half taking a placebo. The researchers were dismayed to find that over the four years, fifty-eight of the placebo-group women died of heart attacks, while seventy-one of the HRT-group women died of heart attacks. In other words, the HRT group had a 23 percent increase in heart attack deaths.[5] Why? One reason may be because the HRT raised their triglyceride levels past the danger point and into the fatal range.

Despite the disappointing results of the HERS study, most conventional doctors point to the dozens of other studies that showed HRT lowers cardiovascular disease rates. What they conveniently overlook is that all of these studies have a fundamental flaw—they are retrospective. Identical groups were not selected for comparison, and that's a scientific no-no. What the studies analyzed were women taking HRT because of their own decision and/or that of their doctors. The control groups were women who decided by themselves not to be on HRT. Menopausal women who aren't in particularly good health—they're overweight or they have diabetes, asthma, or high blood pressure, for instance—often don't use HRT, because they find it makes their problems worse. The women who seek out and continue to use HRT tend to be healthier, slimmer, and more dedicated to lifestyle improvements. In other words, they're less likely to have heart disease with or without HRT.

In fairness, let me say that the standard estrogen/progestin combination used in HRT does indeed lower your total cholesterol, and does raise your level of "good" HDL cholesterol. On the other hand, as mentioned, HRT can sharply elevate that other serious risk factor for heart disease, your triglyceride level. The upward jump could be 30 percent or more.

There is a much better, much more natural way to use hormones to treat the unpleasant effects of menopause—mood swings, vaginal dryness, and the dreaded hot flashes. The latter in particular cries out for a therapy. Some 75 percent of all menopausal women experience these sudden onslaughts of feeling intensely hot and sweating profusely, often for several minutes at a time, whether as an occasional nuisance or as a serious interference with the quality of life. But the hot flash and the rest of the menopause syndrome can be successfully treated with vitanutrients plus a prohormone called natural progesterone. Natural progesterone fights menopausal symptoms, can provide adrenal activity if your body needs it, and protects against the other scourges of older women, osteoporosis and heart disease.

At the Atkins Center, we use natural progesterone made by a compounding pharmacy, or as a rub-on skin cream, combined with vitanutrient supplements. The progesterone cream is easy to use; simply rub about a teaspoon into the skin of your abdomen every night at bedtime for twenty-one days. I usually recommend taking a week off and then starting again. Natural progesterone creams are available over-the-counter at pharmacies and health food stores. But since different products offer different amounts of natural progesterone, be sure you know how much you're getting: Look for products containing 3 percent natural progesterone.

The most important of the vitanutrients to accompany

the cream is folic acid in prescription-strength doses of 30 to 60 mg. Doses this large stimulate natural estrogen production in women and also have an estrogenlike effect that helps to minimize many of the symptoms of menopause. They also consistently stimulate a woman's libido. Here's the problem, though: No one has ever published a study showing exactly what the effects of folic acid are on levels of female hormones, so it's not considered proven medicine.

And because archaic, misogynistic FDA regulations prevent folic acid from being sold in pills larger than 800 mcg without a prescription, you'll have to work with your doctor to be able to take the appropriate dose.

The second menopause-correcting vitanutrient is the mineral boron. This trace mineral has been found to increase estrogen and progesterone levels and to be an effective therapy for osteoporosis, possibly independent of its effect on hormones. I generally prescribe between 10 and 20 mg daily of boron; women notice the difference within a few weeks.

Add to this the most estrogenic of foods, the soybean and its derivatives, and herbs such as black cohosh and others, and you can readily see that there are many elements to choose from to create a successful alternative to HRT.

Most of my patients who take this route find it relieves their menopause symptoms so well that they avoid hormone replacement therapy altogether. Patients can at least lower their doses of the synthetic hormones. That's a desirable endpoint: the smallest amount of estrogen that still controls the woman's symptoms. That at least keeps to a minimum the rise in insulin caused by estrogenic hormones.

BUILDING BONES WITH PROGESTERONE

When HRT enthusiasts learn that the cardiovascular disease mantra is not supportable, they fall back to reciting the osteoporosis mantra. It is true that HRT slows osteoporosis a little, but it does very little to prevent or reverse it. In fact, estrogen loss has less to do with bone loss than you are led to believe. Osteoporosis begins in your late thirties, when your estrogen levels are still normal. By the time you reach your fifties and menopause, you've been slowly losing bone mass for some twenty years.

It's true that after menopause, bone loss accelerates, sometimes to the point of crippling fractures from even the simplest exertion. But it's less the lack of estrogen that causes osteoporosis than it is the lack of progesterone.

Your bones are constantly being remodeled by cells called osteoclasts and osteoblasts. The osteoclasts break down bone; the osteoblasts build it up again. Receptors in the osteoclasts and osteoblasts are sensitive to estrogen and progesterone. We do know from studies that estrogen replacement therapy can slow the breakdown of bone—but only if it's taken during the three to five years around the onset of menopause. After that, estrogen has little—if any—effect on slowing bone loss.

Natural progesterone (the term defines the prohormone rather than the synthetic analogs that are most frequently prescribed) can actually build new bone, enough to balance out or even overcome bone loss. In short, progesterone supplements can help reverse osteoporosis. This works because the bone-building osteoblasts have progesterone receptors, so progesterone stimulates them to get to work creating solid new bone.[6]

Of course, there are expensive drugs with unpleasant side effects that also claim to treat osteoporosis. They work by preventing bone loss. You keep your old bone, rather than going through the natural and normal process of bone remodeling. In the end, I think you're worse off than before, because you're just accumulating old bone, not building new bone. Your bones may be a little denser, but they're no stronger or more resilient.

The majority of Atkins Center patients with decreased bone density have had good results with the natural approach to reversing—not just slowing—osteoporosis. It's safe, it's relatively inexpensive, and it works. The first step is using natural progesterone, folic acid, and boron in the amounts described earlier. A newly available supplement called ipriflavone (IP), made from isoflavones, which are natural plant estrogens, can improve bone density just as estrogen does but without the potential dangers. In fact, just the opposite happens. Estrogen can increase your risk of cancer, while ipriflavone can reduce it.[7]

I recommend taking 600 mg of IP daily, in doses spread out over the day. In addition, you'll need to take supplements of some important vitanutrients such as vitamin D, calcium, magnesium, and strontium, as well as vitamin K. Finally, weight-bearing exercise helps keep your bones strong. Taking a brisk walk for twenty minutes three times a week is a good start in the right direction.

HUMAN GROWTH HORMONE

Should you decide to check out the growing number of antiaging clinics springing up from coast to coast, you will quickly discover that the treatment at many of them is based on the almost routine prescribing and administering of human growth hormone (HGH) and/or substances related to it.

There are two reasons for this phenomenon. One is that patients expect to pay at least $12,000 a year for such treatment, and somewhere in that amount is the possibility of significant profit to the clinic. The second reason is that there can be, and usually is, a very impressive group of beneficial responses to HGH.

These two facts have led to a thriving business opportunity for entrepreneurial doctors, but the facts also carry with them the risk that HGH might be administered to people who really don't need it. In such cases, the treatment could cause a harmful hormonal imbalance.

Having said all that, let me now say that I believe HGH to be one of the most intriguing new hormone-optimizing substances available today. As I explain to you what all the excitement is about, I may have to get a little technical. Please follow along. You'll need this information to understand the tremendous potential of human growth hormone.

As its name suggests, human growth hormone is the hormone that tells your body to grow, to maintain and repair itself. It's an anabolic substance, which means it builds up tissues and functions. In addition, HGH is extremely important for your metabolism—it's involved with just about every aspect of helping your body use energy and remove wastes. It also tells your body when to release fat from body tissues to be burned for energy.

Your endocrine system is a very complex, delicately balanced arrangement of feedback loops, all designed to keep your body running normally and on an even keel. In quantitative terms, HGH is the major hormone put out by your pituitary gland, which is found at the base of your brain and is a key component of the endocrine system. When the pituitary gland gets a message from the other gland-stimulating part of your brain, the hypothalamus, it releases HGH. The HGH then gets carried to your liver, where it stimulates the production of hormonelike substances known as insulin growth factors. The most pertinent of these is insulin growth factor 1 (IGF-1) since it works directly with HGH to regulate your metabolism and promote growth. In fact, we use your levels of IGF-1 to determine how much HGH your pituitary is producing and to judge whether it is sufficient. And IGF-1 can be administered along with HGH, or separately, to achieve nearly identical results.

HGH is released by your pituitary in a cycle of short bursts throughout the day, roughly once every four hours or so. (Your level of IGF-1, however, remains fairly constant throughout the day.) About 70 percent of your HGH production comes at night while you are asleep. Once enough HGH has been released, the hypothalamus sends a second message to your pituitary, using a hormone called somatostatin (also known as GH inhibiting factor), which acts as the messenger telling your pituitary gland to stop making HGH for the moment.

Your production of somatostatin seems to increase with age. That may be one reason your HGH level, which reaches its peak during your teen years, gradually drops off at the rate of about 14 percent per decade. By the time you're age sixty or so, you're making only about 25 percent of the HGH you made when you were twenty.

THE GROWTH HORMONE DEFICIENCY SYNDROME

If your HGH drops a little further or faster than in most people, you can be classified as being deficient in growth hormone. The breakthrough work on growth hormone deficiency (GHD) and on the exciting benefits of HGH was published in 1990 by Dr. Daniel Rudman, who was one of my instructors during my residency at the Goldwater Hospital division of Columbia University. Dr. Rudman's researches defined the criterion for diagnosing growth hormone deficiency as an IGF-1 level below 350 IU. Some 30 percent of apparently healthy sixty-year-old men are below this level. That statistic provides a good guesstimate of how many people should be trying in some way to optimize their IGF-1 level.

Hundreds of scientific studies have been published describing recent findings in GHD.[8] The studies show that the symptoms include an increase in body fat with a simultaneous decrease in lean body mass, muscle bulk, and muscle strength. The studies also show that a loss of body water content, meaning dehydration, is also a feature of GHD, which means that water retention is a possible complication of correcting it. Bone density is decreased in GHD, while fractures from osteoporosis occur more often. Kidney and lung function impairment have been reported as well.

Perhaps the organ most vulnerable to low growth hormone levels is the heart. People with GHD have been found to have elevated risk factors for heart disease: high triglycerides, low HDL, and elevated LDL. This would suggest that insulin resistance, one of the major problems identified in this book, would be found quite often among people with GHD, and in fact, it certainly is.[9]

HGH AS TREATMENT

You have every right to assume that all of the aforementioned manifestations of growth hormone deficiency can be corrected, at least in part, by administering HGH.

But that may be only the start of what HGH can do. Although the idea of using HGH to fight some of the conditions of aging may date back to the work in the 1960s by another of my mentors, Dr. Vladimir Dilman, it was Dr. Rudman's 1990 study, published in the *New England Journal of Medicine*, that opened the floodgates of research on this topic.

Dr. Rudman studied healthy men, albeit frail and elderly, whose IGF-1 levels were below 350 units. He treated twelve of them with a three-times-a-week injected dose of HGH. The study concluded that the effects of six months of HGH on the lean body mass and adipose tissue mass of the men were equivalent in magnitude to the changes incurred during ten to twenty years of aging. The finding set off the HGH revolution.[10]

Among the impressive studies since that time is one showing that HGH or IGF-1, or both, has helped in the treatment of a variety of heart disorders such as congestive heart failure and cardiomyopathy.[11] That means I look at the IGF-1 levels of all my heart patients who also have reduced ability to exert themselves at a normal pace. Part of the treatment plan is to raise their IGF-1 levels to normal.

To me, the area of clinical study that most closely ties HGH into my premise of what causes aging is the work on diabetes. Most of this research has been done using HGH's "kissin' cousin," IGF-1. Quite a few studies confirm that, rather than mimicking the action of insulin, as the name insulinlike growth factor suggests, IGF-1 works to combat insulin *resistance*. That means it lowers both the blood sugar *and* the insulin levels, thus avoiding the need to grasp either horn of the glucose/insulin dilemma. I am particularly excited by a joint study out of the Harvard and North Carolina medical complexes in which both blood sugar and insulin resistance were lowered dramatically with IGF-1.[12] The study was published in the journal *Diabetes*, which is standard reading for all doctors concerned with this disease. All diabetologists should have read it, but just try to find one who will give you HGH or IGF-1.

In addition, HGH has been used successfully to treat fibromyalgia,[13] to overcome wasting in HIV/AIDS and other conditions,[14] and to treat obesity.[15]

THE DOWNSIDE

HGH and IGF-1, although they are natural substances, are prescription drugs, and well they should be. They have real, worrisome side effects. The most striking are water retention, to the point of worsening heart failure even while strengthening the heart; joint pains, including temporomandibular joint problems and carpal tunnel syndrome; increases in heart rate and blood pressure; shortness of breath, headache, and fatigue.

Both my practice experience and my reading of the medical journals convince me that most of these problems are dose-related. They've been reported because of the practice in the research studies of giving a standard dose without frequently checking before-and-after blood levels and lowering the dose as needed. By modifying the protocols to use smaller doses, and by accepting more modest elevations of IGF-1 levels as evidence of improvement, we can avoid virtually all side effects.

HOW TO RAISE YOUR IGF-1

We've come a long way from Dr. Rudman's three-dose-a-week protocol. We have since learned that by synchronizing the administration of the HGH dose with the body's natural nocturnal release of HGH, we can raise the IGF-1 levels with a considerably smaller dose, which also means at considerably less cost. Because your body puts out HGH in brief pulsations, and because most of these occur soon after you fall asleep, I recommend taking a small dose every night at bedtime. A preferable method, suitable for those of you who regularly awaken in the night, is to take a half dose at bedtime and the second half with the first awakening.

This technique not only lets you start with a low dose, it also allows the total dosage to be reduced without sacrificing effectiveness. I usually start my patients with a dosage of 0.0125 units per kilogram of weight per day. (A 220-pound person weighs 100 kg and would therefore start with a nightly dose of 1.25 units. A 176-pound person weighs 80 kg and would therefore take 1 unit daily.) I start patients on HGH in exactly the same way I start them on any other hormone, such as thyroid, that involves considerable risk. I begin with an amount low enough to avoid any dose-related problems, check to see what that accomplishes both with regard to blood levels of IGF-1 and in terms of clinical results and symptom control, and gradually work up the dosage scale until the desired improvement is achieved.

I am inclined to administer treatment when the IGF-1 level is below 350 (below 400 in a younger person). The goal is to bring the IGF-1 level up to 600 (higher in a younger person). I have found, however, that if I can get *all* of the other hormones—DHEA, pregnenolone, androstenedione, testosterone, estrogen, progesterone, and thyroid—into an optimal range, then it is seldom necessary to bring the IGF-1 to a high level.

HOW TO DO IT FOR LESS

There are millions of people who would benefit from raising their HGH level but who find the cost prohibitive. It would seem, from the junk mail I get, that there are thousands of entrepreneurs out there who have recognized that dilemma. Many of them claim to have come up with inexpensive ways to build up your HGH levels without using any HGH at all. This is a worthwhile quest, and one that can be achieved, but not on your own and not with mail-order products.

HGH therapy is not something you can do without a doctor's help, preferably a doctor from the small minority with experience in optimizing hormones. The doctor's role here includes drawing your IGF-1 levels at intervals, writing prescriptions for hormones that can be obtained only by prescription, and evaluating any change in your health status.

Let's look at the most valid and effective treatments that don't require HGH.

DHEA AND HGH

The interaction of DHEA and HGH in your body is a good example of how intricate your endocrine system is. DHEA is manufactured in your body when your hypothalamus tells your pituitary to tell your adrenal glands to make it—the same as with HGH. Because your DHEA and HGH production are controlled in the same way, and because your DHEA production drops as you age just as your HGH production does, there is every reason to believe that the two hormones are very closely linked. And in fact, taking DHEA also makes you produce more IGF-1. It's likely that DHEA makes your body produce more HGH receptor sites on your cells, which would make you more sensitive to the HGH you normally produce. There's no real evidence that DHEA's stimulation of IGF-1 applies to HGH, but there is reason to believe that raising your IGF-1 level gives you many of the same benefits as raising your HGH level.[16]

As you know from the preceding chapter, DHEA has numerous age-defying benefits for your health. In general, it lowers your risk of heart disease, improves your immunity, lifts your mood, and helps prevent cognitive decline. As if those benefits weren't enough, we now know that it helps your body metabolize HGH as well. For all these reasons, I strongly recommend working with your doctor to optimize your DHEA level *before* you embark on an HGH or HGH/IGF-1 program.

MELATONIN AND THE IMPORTANCE OF SLEEP

Since the bulk of your normal HGH production occurs while you are deeply asleep, it's logical to assume that getting a good night's sleep should have a positive impact on your HGH level. The logic goes further. Your pineal gland, another component in your endocrine system, produces a hormone called melatonin. Like HGH, melatonin is mostly secreted at night as your body's way of regulating its sleep-wake cycle. Also like HGH, your production of melatonin naturally declines with age. (Check back to Chapter 9 for some of the other important functions of melatonin.)

Melatonin helps you fall asleep and stay asleep. Many people, especially those over age sixty or so, have trouble falling asleep precisely because their melatonin levels are low. They wake up frequently during the night and in general don't sleep very deeply. That also means they're not releasing as much HGH as they would if they slept better.

Research into the connection between melatonin and HGH is still in the early stages, so we can't say for sure that taking melatonin will increase your HGH production. But it's logical. After all, the melatonin will almost certainly help you sleep well—and naturally, without dangerous and possibly addictive drugs, and with no hangover effect. And a good night's sleep can't help but maximize your HGH production.

Since the dosage of melatonin varies enormously from one person to the next, you'll need to experiment a bit to find the dose that works for you. Start with 0.5 to 1 mg taken about an hour before your normal bedtime. You should start to feel drowsy about half an hour after taking the melatonin. If a smaller dose doesn't do much for you, increase it gradually to 3 mg (considered a standard dose), and if that fails, move up to 5 or even 10 mg until you notice results. Doses up to 20 mg a day are generally safe. But don't take melatonin if you are taking steroid drugs.

STIMULATING HGH: THYROID FUNCTION, AMINO ACIDS

Just as optimizing sleep can optimize your production of HGH, there are other functions it also helps to enhance in order to boost your level of HGH.

I'll be telling you about the importance of your thyroid gland soon. For now, let me just emphasize that optimizing thyroid function may help make your existing

HGH supply go further, whether it's natural HGH or supplements.

Similarly, several amino acids stimulate your body to produce HGH, while some others may have a similar but less pronounced effect. The one we know most about is arginine, an essential amino acid—that is, one your body can't create for itself. Arginine has been shown to increase your secretion of growth hormone by blocking the effect of somatostatin, the hormone that tells your pituitary gland to stop making growth hormone.[17]

Right now, the problem is that studies of the oral dosages needed to have any effect show a wide variation.[18] This may be considerably less of a problem than it seems, however. Arginine is widely used as a treatment for angina pectoris in dosages of 15 grams. I know from my own experience with angina patients and from the research on the subject that arginine causes virtually no side effects at dosages that high. I have no problem recommending doses of between 5 and 15 g to see if it causes an improvement in IGF-1 levels.

The nonessential amino acid ornithine is manufactured in your body from arginine. It is so similar chemically to arginine that it has a very similar effect in the body. The drawback is that while ornithine is roughly twice as effective as arginine for the same dose, it's also twice as expensive. As with arginine, the most effective doses are still not really known. For that reason, I prefer to have my patients use arginine and skip the ornithine.

Lysine, another essential amino acid, works synergistically with arginine to boost your HGH output, but only if you're in your twenties. The combination doesn't do anything for older adults, even at doses as high as 6 g each.[19]

A more promising approach is glutamine, the most abundant amino acid in your body. Glutamine is considered conditionally essential, in other words, you can ordinarily easily synthesize all you need from your food. In times of stress or injury, however, glutamine synthesis may be impaired. Because glutamine is the primary fuel for the intestines, I have long used it as a very valuable treatment for patients with such digestive tract ailments as Crohn's disease and colitis. Glutamine also stimulates your body to release growth hormone.[20] It's readily available in pills, capsules, or a tasteless powder at any health food store. I suggest taking at least 2 g daily at bedtime. Glutamine has the added benefits of being safe and inexpensive.

A number of manufacturers now offer arginine and other HGH-stimulating amino acids in combination formulas. Some also offer a sublingual spray that is said to give the same effect with a smaller dose that is absorbed directly into your bloodstream. Be skeptical about purchasing these products—many don't really have a large enough dose to be useful. The advertising is sometimes misleading, suggesting that the sprays contain HGH. They do not. HGH is available only with a doctor's prescription.

HYDERGINE AND HGH

Of all the drugs that raise HGH, the only one I would consider prescribing for a patient with a serious HGH deficiency is Hydergine. My European colleagues have long used it with good results for improving cognitive ability in their elderly patients.[21] It's also often touted as a "smart drug" that can increase your brain power.

Studies show that Hydergine is quite safe, with a low risk of side effects. There haven't been any long-term studies of its effectiveness for raising HGH levels, but in the short run it definitely helps.

PUMPING UP HGH

Exercise of any sort stimulates the release of HGH. Any form of exercise is better than none, but weight training seems to give the most dramatic increases in HGH. I realize that this is not the form of exercise best suited to many people. You'll have to join a gym and work with an instructor to learn how to use free weights and weight-training machines properly.

If you don't want to complicate your life that much, you can still get an increase in your HGH levels from taking a brisk walk, riding a bicycle or exercise bike, doing calisthenics, or undertaking any other form of exercise that you enjoy and can do regularly.

DIET AND HGH

Growth hormone deficiency is made considerably worse if you are overweight, because obesity lowers your level of human growth hormone every bit as much as advancing age does. The heavier you are, the less HGH you have; the less body fat you have, the more HGH you will have.[22]

But even if you're not obese, you can boost your HGH levels through diet. And you won't be surprised to read that the best diet for doing that while also improving your overall health is a low-carbohydrate, high-protein diet.

And speaking of diet, it's time to address the subject of fat.

14

GOOD FATS AND *REALLY* BAD FATS

I can't go any further into this book without giving you a clear understanding of the crucial role fats play in your age-defying diet. Fats? Yes, fats, the four-letter word we've become terrified to utter—and of course terrified to eat. The medical establishment, with pronouncements that have been misleading at best and downright harmful at worst, has frightened many of us into avoiding dietary fats altogether. We end up eating far too little of the fats that can help our health, and far too high a percentage of the fats that can harm us.

For there are both good fats and bad fats—essential fats that you need to live and stay healthy and help you defy the effects of aging, bad fats that speed the aging process, and one type, the trans fats, that you most certainly should avoid if you are to live your maximum life span in good health.

In this chapter, we'll look at exactly what fats are and do, why you need to consume some and how best to do so, and why you must avoid others. But first, I want to set the record straight. The American public has been fed so much blubber about fat that the entire subject has become obscure. To make it possible for the truth about fats to come through, therefore, my first task is to clear up the mystery and misinformation that have so misled people.

SATURATION POINT

It all has to do with the great fallacy long perpetrated on an unsuspecting nation—the dead-wrong heart-diet hypothesis. The biggest confusion concerns the main types of *dietary* fats (as distinguished from the organic compounds in our bodies): saturated, monounsaturated, and polyunsaturated. Years of agribusiness propaganda have led people to believe that saturated fats must be avoided at all costs and that the more unsaturated a fat is, the better. Let's look more closely at exactly what that means.

As I'll explain in a bit more detail a few paragraphs down, all fats are chains made up mostly of carbon and hydrogen atoms, with some oxygen molecules attached at the end. The carbon atoms are the backbone of the chain. If all the carbon atoms in the chain are bound to as many hydrogen atoms as they can hold, the fat is said to be saturated. Animal fats such as butter and lard are saturated; so are some vegetable oils such as coconut oil and palm oil. These fats are generally solid at room temperature.

If some hydrogen atoms are missing from the chain, the carbon atoms fill the gap by linking up with double chemical bonds, and the fat is said to be unsaturated. Monounsaturated fats have one extra carbon double bond; polyunsaturated fats have two or more double carbon bonds. Unsaturated fats such as olive oil, corn oil, and other vegetable oils are liquid at room temperature. Olive oil and nut oils are very high in monounsaturated fats; corn oil and safflower oil are very high in polyunsaturated fats.

Saturated fats from animal foods such as meat and dairy products contain large amounts of cholesterol, which, as you well know by this time, is a type of waxy fat produced in the liver of animals, including humans, and used for many crucial metabolic functions. Eating foods high in saturated fat from animals therefore means you're also eating foods high in cholesterol, which in turn will raise the amount of cholesterol in your blood. For decades now, the prevailing wisdom has been that eating foods high in saturated fats and thus in cholesterol inevitably leads to clogged arteries, and that eating foods high in polyunsaturated fats keeps your arteries clear. It's the simplistic message you hear constantly from every quarter—and it's wrong.

What often gets forgotten in discussions of fats is that all dietary fats actually contain a mixture of saturated and unsaturated fats. Butter, for instance, is 66 percent saturated fat; the rest is mostly monounsaturated fat. Corn oil is 62 percent polyunsaturated fat, 25 percent monounsaturated fat, and 13 percent saturated fat. The fat you store in your body is almost entirely saturated, and it's saturated fat the medical establishment has warned us all to reduce or avoid.

The thing that continually astonishes me about the recommendation to avoid saturated fat is not that it is based on practically no solid evidence, although that is bewildering enough. Rather, what really amazes me is how the medical establishment is so blinkered that it ignores the strong evidence in exactly the opposite direction.

The study your doctor is most likely to cite in favor of the saturated fat–heart disease hypothesis is the famous Framingham Heart Study, which has been following the diets and health of a large group of people living in Framingham, Massachusetts, since the 1940s. Here's what Dr. William Castelli, the director of the study, had to say about it in 1992: "In Framingham, Massachusetts, the more saturated fat one ate, the more cholesterol one ate, the more calories one ate, the lower people's serum cholesterol. . . . We found that the people who ate the most cholesterol, ate the most saturated fat, ate the most calories weighed the least and were the most physically active."[1]

More recently, in 1997, there was a major article in the well-regarded *European Heart Journal* titled "The Low Fat/Low Cholesterol Diet Is Ineffective." The article went on to review all the major studies of diet and heart disease over the last twenty years to prove exactly what the title said it would.[2] That article was followed in 1998 by another meta-analysis of the role of saturated and polyunsaturated fatty acids in cardiovascular disease. The conclusion again was that serious questions have arisen about the role of dietary saturated fats in causing heart disease, and the supposed role of polyunsaturated fatty acids in preventing it.[3]

In case all that's not enough to make you start asking your doctor some hard questions, consider two other recent studies. The first looked at the cholesterol levels of stroke patients and compared them to cholesterol levels in healthy people. They found that high cholesterol was associated with a higher risk of ischemic stroke, which happens when the flow of blood to the brain is blocked. The patients who had hemorrhagic strokes, which cause bleeding *into* the brain, had low cholesterol, below 180 mg. Their risk of stroke was twice that of someone with cholesterol of 230 mg. The reason is that cholesterol is crucial for maintaining the integrity of your blood vessels. Without it, the blood vessels can leak, sometimes catastrophically.[4]

Even more telling is a 1999 study that shows how a low-fat diet actually increases your chances of heart disease. In this study, 238 healthy men spent several weeks eating a diet that took 40 percent of its calories from fat, and then spent an equal amount of time eating a diet that derived only 20 to 24 percent of its calories from fat. You might think that while the men were on the low-fat diet their blood lipid profile would improve. In fact, just the opposite happened. About a third of the men who ate the low-fat diet showed some worrisome lipid changes. They started making more small, dense LDL particles, more triglycerides, and less HDL cholesterol.[5]

Despite all this, your conventional doctor is probably still recommending that you eat margarine instead of butter. What he or she is really doing is ensuring that you will be a lifelong patient. Margarine, the fat that agribusiness spends millions a year to advertise, is the worst fat of them all. Why? Because margarine is a trans fat, a fabricated food formed by taking a vegetable oil like corn oil, stripping off the essential fatty acids, and processing what's left by forcing additional hydrogen atoms into it. The result is a fat that's more saturated, which means it is soft or solid at room temperature.

Trans fats, also known as partially hydrogenated vegetable oils, are completely unnatural. Even worse, trans fats are so widely used in the average American diet that they have largely replaced the essential fatty acids in their natural forms. I'll go into the details of why trans fats are so dangerous toward the end of this chapter. For now, let's turn to essential fatty acids and see why, as the name implies, you absolutely need them.

THE GOOD FATS

Despite what the American Heart Association and others would have you believe, you need fat to live and stay healthy. You especially need what are known as essential fatty acids. Note the use of the word "essential." In scientific as well as everyday usage, essential means just that: something you have to have. Just as vitamins by definition are substances your body can't manufacture and that must therefore be obtained from your food— and from supplements, as needed—so too must the essential fatty acids come from your diet. Unfortunately, they often don't. I believe that the essential fatty acids are the primary nutrient missing from the American diet. Let's look at them a little more closely.

Any fat molecule is made from a chain of carbon atoms bound to hydrogen atoms. At the tail end of the chain—the omega end—is a carbon atom attached to two oxygen atoms, which is what makes the fat an acid. Your body needs to manufacture twenty different fatty acids in all, and it must manufacture them from just two *essential* fatty acids: omega-3, also known as linolenic acid, and omega-6, also known as linoleic acid.

The omega-3 family of fatty acids can be further subdivided into three groups: alpha-linolenic acid (LNA), eicosapentaenoic acid (EPA), and docosahexanoic acid (DHA). In general, omega-3s are found in the leaves and seeds of many plants, in egg yolks, and in such cold-water ocean fish as herring, tuna, cod, and mackerel. LNA is found in plant foods, especially nuts, soybeans, canola oil, and flaxseed oil. EPA and DHA are found in fish oil.

Similarly, the omega-6 family of fatty acids falls into three groups: gamma-linoleic acid (GLA), arachidonic acid, and dihomo-linoleic acid. Of the three, only GLA and, to a lesser extent, arachidonic acid are really relevant to our discussion here. GLA is found in dark green leafy vegetables, egg yolks, and whole grains and seeds. It's very abundant in the seeds of some plants, especially borage and evening primrose, that aren't commonly eaten.

A third group of fatty acids, the omega-9s, isn't essential, but it is extremely helpful. The most widely used source of omega-9 fatty acid, also known as oleic acid, is olive oil. Omega-9s are also found in peanut oil, sesame oil, nut oils, and avocados and avocado oil.

WHAT ESSENTIAL FATTY ACIDS DO

Your body uses essential fatty acids for a number of important functions. First and foremost, they're used to make eicosanoids and prostaglandins, short-lived, hormonelike substances that regulate many activities in your body. Among other things, eicosanoids and prostaglandins control your blood pressure and your body temperature; regulate inflammation, swelling, and pain; and are involved in blood clotting, allergic reactions, and the making of other hormones.

As your body makes the different eicosanoids and prostaglandins, it's important that the two types of fatty acids remain in balance. That's because your body uses mostly omega-3s to make some of these substances and mostly omega-6s to make others. Think of the two fatty acids as the brake and accelerator pedals in a car—you need both pedals to drive. If you keep your foot on just one or the other, you're driving unsafely; you need to apply both pedals judiciously, each for its special purpose.

But in the American diet today, we've got our foot stuck on the essential fatty acids accelerator, and we're heading for a crash. The introduction of vegetable oils made from corn, peanuts, and other sources has led to a serious imbalance in the amounts of omega-3 and omega-6 fatty acids in our diet. In general, humans need to take in at least 2 to 3 percent of their fat as omega-6 fatty acids and at least 1 to 1.5 percent as omega-3s. Put another way, you need about twice as much omega-6 as omega-3 fatty acids. Unfortunately, the modern American diet has this balance seriously distorted, to the point where we eat many times more omega-6 fatty acids.

Historically, in the days before refined vegetable oils, people got their essential fatty acids from whole grains, nuts, vegetables, and egg yolks. Today, the average American consumes large amounts of refined corn, soy, safflower, and canola oil, which are extra high in omega-6 fatty acids, and eats relatively little omega-3 fatty acids in the form of fish, egg yolks, nuts and nut oils, unrefined vegetable oils, and whole grains. The resulting imbalance, along with the widespread use of trans fats, is strongly implicated, in my opinion and in the opinion of many others, in the epidemic levels of heart disease, cancer, inflammatory ailments, autoimmune illnesses, and other chronic, degenerative diseases of the twentieth century. Rebalancing your intake of these essential fatty acids is crucial to the age-defying diet.

OMEGA-3s AND YOUR HEART

Let's take heart disease as one very clear example of the value of omega-3s. As early as 1908, researchers noted that heart disease was unknown among Greenland natives, even though these people subsisted almost entirely on meat. The same lack of heart disease was found when the Greenlanders were studied again in the 1930s. In the decade of the 1970s, there was not a single death from heart disease among a group of 3,000 natives. To this day, heart disease is very rare among Greenlanders who eat a traditional diet.

Why? The native Greenlander diet consists of almost nothing but the meat and blubber from seals and small whales. Because these mammals feed exclusively on cold-water fish, their flesh is very high in omega-3 fatty acids, which in turn confer their protection on the humans who eat them.[6] Native Greenlanders who move to Denmark and begin eating a typical European diet quickly develop levels of heart disease comparable to their Danish neighbors.

The benefits of omega-3 fatty acids for your heart are extremely well documented. They lower triglycerides and LDL cholesterol, discourage arterial plaque, act as an anticoagulant to prevent dangerous blood clots, reduce high blood pressure, prevent strokes, and perhaps most important of all, prevent sudden death from cardiac arrhythmias.

I could back up all these statements with a discussion of literally hundreds of studies, many of them showing a significant lowering of the major heart risk factor, high triglycerides, but let's look at just a few of the more recent. In a study of more than 11,000 Italian patients recovering from heart attacks, the omega-3 fatty acids in fish oil made a significant difference in their recovery. Over a three-and-a-half-year period, daily supplementation with 1,000 mg of fish oil was associated with an overall 10 percent reduced risk for death, fatal or nonfatal heart attack, or stroke, compared with patients who didn't receive the supplements. The researchers believe that fish oil's ability to prevent dangerous heart rhythm problems is what made the difference.[7]

This study backs up similar results that were obtained from the well-known 1989 DART (Diet and Reinfarction Trial) study of men who had already had a heart attack. The ones who ate fish at least twice a week had a 29 percent decline in death from any cause compared to the men who didn't change their diets.[8]

Perhaps most important of all, eating fish at least once a week can cut your risk of sudden cardiac death in half. This is borne out by results from the ongoing Physicians' Health Study. Researchers have been following the diets and health of more than 20,000 male doctors since 1983. Between 1983 and 1994, 133 of the physicians died from sudden cardiac death. The ones who ate fish at least once a week, however, had a 52 percent lower risk of such a death. Again, the research points to omega-3 as providing protection against fatal heart arrhythmias.[9]

PREVENTING CANCER WITH ESSENTIAL FATTY ACIDS

Just as eating fish just once or twice a week can sharply reduce your chances of dying from heart disease, so too can it reduce your chances of dying from cancer. A major study in Italy that compared 10,000 cancer patients to 8,000 patients with other problems showed that those who ate two or more servings of fish a week had a much lower risk for specific cancers compared to those who ate fish less than once a week. To be precise, the fish eaters' rates of esophageal, stomach, colon, rectal, and pancreatic cancers were 30 to 50 percent lower.[10]

OTHER BENEFITS OF ESSENTIAL FATTY ACIDS

The benefits of essential fatty acids go considerably beyond heart attack and cancer prevention. Complementary practitioners have long known that fish oil is a valuable treatment for rheumatoid arthritis and other autoimmune diseases such as lupus, multiple sclerosis, and scleroderma. At the Atkins Center, we use fish oil as a very effective treatment for Crohn's disease, colitis, and other inflammatory bowel diseases.[11] We also use fish oil to treat such skin problems as atopic eczema and psoriasis.

Fish oil has also recently been shown to help prevent osteoporosis by inhibiting the production of a prostaglandin that limits bone growth. Adding fish oil to the diet also enhances the activity of insulinlike growth factor (IGF), a substance closely related to human growth hormone. Because IGF stimulates your body to grow and remodel bone, raising your level of it helps prevent osteoporosis.[12]

I've used fish oil as a treatment for mood disorders, particularly depression, with good results for many years. Recently, my approach was borne out by a study of thirty patients receiving standard drug therapy for manic depression. Half of the patients took fish oil capsules; the other half took olive oil capsules. Most of the patients on fish oil maintained or improved their mental condition. Most of the patients on olive oil didn't.[13]

INSTEAD OF DRUGS

Apart from fish oil, another important benefit of the essential fatty acids comes from altering your balance of omega-3s and omega-6s to affect your production of eicosanoids and prostaglandins. Since these chemical messengers control pain and inflammation in your body, altering the balance to produce more of the desirable eicosanoids and prostaglandins and fewer of the undesirable ones can lessen your reliance on pain-killing drugs.

In fact, inhibiting production of prostaglandins is exactly what the two most widely used drugs in medicine do—steroids, and nonsteroidal anti-inflammatories like aspirin. Both inhibit your production of all prostaglandins, good and bad. How much more sensible it would be to alter only the prostaglandins that are harmful, and to do it without powerful drugs and their harmful side effects.

THE OMEGA-6s AND GLA

And let's not forget the omega-6 family. Perhaps the most valuable benefit of omega-6 fatty acids is realized when they are transformed into gamma-linolenic acid (GLA). You need GLA for making one of your body's most important natural ways of fending off degenerative diseases, prostaglandin E_1. The problem is that the enzyme you use to convert the omega-6s to GLA is often in very short supply in your body. In part, that's because you just naturally make less of it as you get older. In part, it may also be due to a diet high in sugar and partially hydrogenated vegetable oils, which tends to suppress your production of the enzyme. The result is a serious shortage of GLA and an increased risk of disease.

But supplements can help. At the Atkins Center, we use GLA in the form of borage oil or evening primrose oil to help treat a variety of problems. The most common use is for relieving the symptoms of premenstrual tension that are often associated with premenstrual syndrome, or PMS. The results are generally remarkable. After three months of treatment at 300 mg a day, most women find that such symptoms of PMS as irritability, cramps, and breast tenderness disappear.

We also find GLA highly effective for treating arthritis. Indeed, this is the best documented of all the uses of GLA.[14] GLA is very helpful for relieving the joint swelling, morning stiffness, and pain that come with arthritis. It's also useful for some other common problems, such as nerve damage from diabetes and high cholesterol.

GETTING THE BENEFITS OF FATTY ACIDS

You can gain the benefits of the fatty acids through diet, supplements, and a combination of the two—for example, fish for dinner and fish oil as a supplement.

For starters, just by following the age-defying diet I outline in this book, you will remove the two major causes of deficiency in essential fatty acids. First, you'll be eating far fewer refined carbohydrates and far more eggs, fish, and dark green leafy vegetables. That means you'll naturally be getting a lot more omega-3 and omega-6 fatty acids from your diet. Second, you'll be replacing the worthless trans fats in your diet with unrefined natural vegetable oils such as flaxseed oil, olive oil, and the oils of other seeds and nuts. This too will naturally raise your levels of the essential fatty acids and restore them to a more natural balance.

Recent results from the ongoing Nurses' Health Study show how easy it is to add omega-3s to your diet—and what a difference it can make. The study tracked the diets and health of more than 76,000 women for more than ten years. During that time, 232 of the women died, while 597 developed heart disease. One of the major dietary differences between the women who stayed healthy and those who didn't was the amount of oil-based salad dressing consumed. Mayonnaise, creamy salad dressing, and oil and vinegar dressings are all, of course, rich in omega-3, and they served as the most common dietary source of omega-3 in the study. The women who ate these dressings five or more times a week definitely had healthier hearts than the ones who ate them only rarely.[15]

Here's an excellent example of how fat-phobia actually leads inexorably to more heart disease rather than less. Many people, in their dread of fat of any kind, opt for fat-free salad dressings, even though there's plenty of firm evidence to show that they should be pouring on dressings rich in these valuable oils instead. You can make your salad dressing even more valuable by adding a tablespoon of flaxseed oil to it. This mild, almost flavorless oil is a very rich source of the essential omega-3, alpha-linolenic acid.

Another good way to get the age-defying heart protection of omega-3s from your diet is by eating more fish, especially cold-water fish like salmon, cod, mackerel, sardines, herring, and bluefish. There's no easy way to determine how often you need to eat fish to make a real change in your omega-3 level, but even eating it just twice a week has been shown in several studies to make a measurable difference in successful outcomes. Even if you add fish to your diet, I still recommend taking fish oil supplements as well.

Just about the only way you can get extra GLA is by taking capsules of evening primrose oil, borage seed oil, or black currant seed oil. Of the three, the most inexpensive is borage oil, but the jury is still out on which is the best choice.

To make sure you're getting all the essential fatty acids you need in the right proportions, I recommend that the average person take a mixture of fish oil, flax-seed oil, and borage seed oil, providing 400 mg each of the omega-3 fatty acid ALA, EPA, DHA, and the omega-6 fatty acid GLA—one to three times daily.

Like all oils, essential fatty acids are vulnerable to oxidation, even after you swallow them. You certainly don't want any extra oxidation happening inside your blood vessels. What stops it? Vitamin E and selenium. One reason the seal-eating Greenlanders have such low cholesterol levels is that seal oil turns out to be naturally very high in vitamin E and selenium. In fact, Greenlanders who live in the traditional hunting community of Siorapaluk, the northernmost settlement in the world, have selenium levels ten to twenty times higher than Europeans or Americans. Free radicals don't have a chance with these people.[16] To get the most benefit from your essential fatty acid supplements, I strongly recommend taking them with a 400 IU capsule of natural vitamin E plus selenium.

ADDING ESSENTIAL FATTY ACIDS TO YOUR DIET

Adding essential fatty acids to your diet is an important component of the age-defying diet. And it's easy to do. Just substitute unrefined vegetable oils that are mostly monounsaturated or high in omega-3 fatty acids for the mostly polyunsaturated cooking you may now be using. In other words, if corn oil is your usual cooking oil, replace it with olive oil, nut oil, or flaxseed oil.

Olive oil is ideal for high-temperature cooking such as sautéing. It is also excellent for salad dressings and homemade mayonnaise. Flaxseed oil is a mild, almost flavorless oil that is extremely high in alpha-linolenic acid. Add a spoonful to salad dressings and the like, but don't heat it—you'll oxidize the ALA. Nut oils, such as walnut oil, add a rich flavor to salad dressings.

Commercial cooking oils have been heavily processed at high temperatures in harsh chemicals, so a lot of their nutritional value has been destroyed long before they end up in your shopping cart. I strongly urge you to purchase cold-pressed, unrefined cooking oils at your health food store. To prevent oxidation, the oils should be stored in the refrigerator in opaque bottles.

Another good way to get extra omega-3s in your diet is to go a little nuts. By that I mean to eat a handful of walnuts, macadamias, almonds, pecans, hazelnuts, or even peanuts (which technically are legumes, not nuts) every day. Going back to the Nurses' Health Study, researchers recently found that the women who ate nuts regularly had a 32 percent lower risk of suffering a nonfatal heart attack and were 39 percent less likely to die of a heart attack than those who consumed nuts rarely or never.[17] The amount of nuts needed to provide the protection was low, only five ounces a week.

Similar results from the Physicians' Health Study suggest that frequent nut consumption has the same benefits for men. The fatty acids in the nuts help to lower LDL cholesterol and triglycerides while leaving HDL cholesterol at the same level or even raising it. I especially recommend the nuts high in monounsaturated fat such as macadamias, hazelnuts, and pecans. Peanuts are good too, but avoid most commercial peanut butters, which can be loaded with trans fats and extra sugar.

THE MEDITERRANEAN DIET

All this talk of oils and fish and nuts brings us directly to the benefits—alleged and real—of the Mediterranean diet. As you doubtless know from reading all the reports about it in the press, the heart-protective Mediterranean diet is said to be what the natives of Greece and Italy eat. It is high in fresh fruits and vegetables, whole grains, fish, olive oil, and red wine. The nutritional establishment has seized on the fact that red meat, butter, and dairy products are relatively infrequent components of the Mediterranean diet and have proclaimed this as proof that a high-carbohydrate, low-fat diet is indeed the healthiest way to eat.

What they don't quite see is that the two things that make the Mediterranean diet healthy are the dearth of refined carbohydrates and the high amount of essential fatty acids in it from fish fat, olive oil, and nut oils. In fact, a recent study has shown that the monounsaturated fats in the Mediterranean diet help protect you against age-related memory loss. The higher your consumption of olive oil, which is a very rich source of monounsaturated oleic acid (omega-9 fatty acid), the better protected you are.[18]

TRANS FATS: THE WORST

What makes trans fats so dangerous? First, we need to know what they are.

Also known as partially hydrogenated oils, trans fats are polyunsaturated vegetable oils that have been processed to make them solid at room temperature. They are used extensively in processed foods, especially baked goods. To see what I mean, go to the cookie aisle of your supermarket and read the ingredients list on just about any package, even the so-called whole-grain breads and the super-premium cookies. Partially hydrogenated vegetable oil is sure to be in the top three or four ingredients, right after the enriched white flour. You'll also find this stuff in all sorts of other prepared foods, including prepared entrees, mayo, salad dressings, candy bars, potato chips, and lots more. And of course, margarine, even the low-fat kind, is by definition nothing but a stick or tub of trans fats.

Any food fried in polyunsaturated oil—the french fries at your favorite fast-food restaurant, for example—is basically just cooked in trans fats, probably made from soybean oil. Whenever you deep-fry foods in corn, safflower, peanut, and other common oils, you're creating trans fats, and the foods you've cooked are far unhealthier for you— and more fattening—than food fried in such saturated fats as lard, tallow, or palm oil. In fact, if you need a second reason, beyond sugar and flour, why Americans today are fatter than ever, trans fats are it.

What makes these molecular misfits so very dangerous, however, is the way they raise your LDL cholesterol, triglyceride, and lipoprotein(a) levels and lower your HDL cholesterol—the worst possible combination of lipid changes and the surest markers we have of almost certain cardiovascular disease sooner rather than later in life.[19] Instead of wrongly blaming saturated fat from animal foods for atherosclerosis, the finger should be pointed straight at trans fats.*

Trans fats not only displace the natural fats and oils that provide essential fatty acids, they also block your

---

*In fact, it was all the way back in 1956 that researcher Dr. Ancel Keys claimed that the trans fats in partially hydrogenated vegetable oils were the culprits. The edible oils industry put a quick stop to that claim and quickly shifted the blame to animal fats. Dr. Keys went on to author the famous/ infamous 1966 Seven Countries study that provided the "proof" that high saturated fat consumption in a population correlates directly to high rates of heart disease. This study, felt to be deeply flawed by the selective citation of nations chosen to prove the point, has since become the touchstone of the fat-phobic public policy now being foisted on Americans.

uptake and use of the essential fatty acids you do manage to take in. What happens then? The trans fats end up being deposited in parts of your cell membranes that should really be filled by essential fatty acids. This quite literally gums up the works. Aside from weakening the integrity of the cell membranes, you also have trouble making the enzyme that converts essential fatty acids into the other fatty acids you need.[20]

In addition, trans fats aggravate the problem I consider the most responsible for shortening life: They make you put out more insulin than normal in response to blood glucose, while making your red blood cells less responsive to insulin.[21]

The medical establishment, backed up by the massive American food-processing industry, has been ignoring the glaring dangers of trans fats ever since the first evidence was published in the 1950s. Numerous other studies have been published since then, particularly by the distinguished fat researcher Mary G. Enig, Ph.D. Recently, even the establishment medical press has published major studies pointing out the dangers of trans fats and even admitting that earlier recommendations to eat margarine instead of butter were foolish.[22] The word still hasn't seeped out to all conventional doctors, however—or if it has, they've decided to ignore it. Most still parrot the party line that saturated fats are the culprit.

Don't believe it for a minute. Trans fats are a major reason why heart disease was practically nonexistent before 1910, when margarine was introduced as a cheap and "healthy" substitute for butter. Crisco, a partially hydrogenated vegetable shortening, was introduced in 1911. By 1950, annual butter consumption dropped from eighteen pounds per person to just ten pounds per person, but margarine consumption went up from two pounds per person to eight. In 1909, the average American consumed fewer than two grams a day of liquid vegetable oils. In 1993, that number had jumped to over thirty grams. Combine the switch from animal fats to liquid vegetable oils with the fact that refined carbohydrate intake escalated at the same time and you have a convincing explanation for the increase in heart attack deaths from 3,000 in 1930 to half a million just thirty years later.

Today, as results from the Nurses' Health Study make clear, your risk of a heart attack is nearly double the average if you get just 2 percent of your calories from the trans fats in doughnuts, french fries, margarine, and similar foods. Unfortunately, 2 percent of your calories from trans fats is almost certainly on the low side for a typical American today. Fat expert Mary Enig believes the typical intake of trans fats is much higher; in fact, based on solid evidence, she believes that about 11 percent of the total fat in the diet of the average American today is trans fat. That works out to be closer to 4 percent of the average American's total daily calories[23]—a number that doesn't surprise me in the least.

According to the U.S. Department of Agriculture, potato chips, which are nothing but a vehicle for delivering trans fat into the diet, are officially a vegetable. The two most popular "vegetables" among teenagers are potato chips and french fries. The Agriculture Department also says that among teens thirteen to eighteen years old, chips and fries make up 31 percent of their total vegetable consumption. These eating habits don't improve much with age. Among adults age nineteen to thirty, chips and fries make up 22 to 25 percent of total vegetable consumption.

Trans fats are ubiquitous and insidious, yet the amounts in prepared foods aren't required to be listed on the labels. Many fast foods are practically nothing *but* trans fats. A large order of fries at a fast-food restaurant, for instance, could easily contain nearly 7 grams of trans fats, but the restaurant proudly proclaims that the fries are cholesterol free! Fortunately, there is a strong movement afoot at the FDA to force manufacturers to list the amount of trans fats on their labels separately from the amount of saturated fat. I hope that the adoption of this regulation will happen soon. If and when it does, it will be a rare instance of the FDA showing some common sense.

I've learned over the years that most of my patients and readers have plenty of common sense—that's why they're interested in their health. And it's common sense, of course, to do everything you can to avoid getting sick. In the next chapter, I'll tell you about ways to boost your immunity.

15

BUILDING YOUR IMMUNITY

Throughout your lifetime, you are constantly being exposed to infectious disease. Indeed, well into the early decades of the twentieth century, infectious diseases were a leading cause of shortened life spans.

But throughout history, there were always individuals who did not fall victim to the plagues and epidemics that were destroying the people around them. The most logical explanation for this, and certainly the most hopeful, is that these people naturally had greater immune system defenses. And while the major message of this book is that diet is central to defying age and preventing many chronic illnesses, the truth is that diet may not be enough. To triumph over the effects of aging, we must also deal with a variety of chronic relapsing pathogens capable of causing serious illness and capable of coming back once "eradicated," whenever our defenses are down.

Moreover, you've probably noticed that you're more likely to get sick when you're under stress. That's because stress produces the hormone cortisol, and cortisol can slow your immune system or shut it down altogether by blocking your production of chemical messengers. In earlier times—say, a hundred thousand years ago when life was simpler—no lasting harm derived from shutting down your immune system occasionally while your body's energies were diverted to fighting off a cave bear. At the start of the twenty-first century, however, life is lived at a consistently high level of stress, and it's quite likely that our cortisol levels, which rise naturally as we get older in any event, are continuously high—with a correspondingly depressing effect on our immunity.

What is the immune system? How does it work? Your body's primary defense against invading pathogens starts with your skin and your epithelial cells—the linings of your organs, including your respiratory and intestinal tracts. If these are weak, harmful infectious agents can enter more easily. Should an infectious agent make it past your epithelial defenses, your internal defense systems take over, and various white blood cells, antibodies, and chemical messengers go to work to keep the pathogens from causing damage. As yet another line of defense, all the parts of your immune system are on constant patrol to detect not just invading pathogens but also damaged and potentially cancerous cells within your body.

Obviously, you want all components of this elaborate system to be as strong as possible for as long as possible. This chapter will help you strengthen and boost your immune system so that you can bring to bear the most powerful immune defenses possible and defy the effects of aging. What you eat can play a central role in this, but you must also pay careful attention to vitanutrients and lifestyle to achieve resilience as well as strength in your immune system.

Let's start with diet—to make sure we're avoiding foods that lower our immunity and eating those foods that strengthen and enhance our immune defenses.

EATING FOR IMMUNITY

Whenever I put a patient on a low-carbohydrate, high-protein diet, I schedule follow-up visits, including one for a few months later. At that visit, my patients almost always say things like, "Doctor, I haven't been sick once since I went on your diet" or "Doctor, that nagging infection I had cleared up just a few days after I started the diet." I'm never surprised to hear this. Indeed, the only surprise would be if someone told me the opposite.

There's no question that the age-defying diet in this book improves your immunity, but how? Your immune system is a very complex and interconnected arrangement of many different kinds of immune cells and chemical messengers, including hormones, eicosanoids, and enzymes. To function efficiently, the system needs a good supply of high-quality protein and crucial vitanutrients. That's why malnourished populations are so susceptible to epidemics of infectious disease: Their immune systems are weakened by poor nutrition, especially from a lack of protein.

If you take in all the protein and vitanutrients your immune system needs, however, and still also take in high levels of carbohydrates, you won't get the full benefit of increased immunity. High carbohydrates are almost certain to lead to high levels of glucose in your blood, which in turn will cause you to release large amounts of insulin—and high levels of insulin can severely depress your immune system. By controlling your blood sugar and insulin levels, and keeping them as low as possible, you keep your immune system at a high level of readiness.

Sugar in itself also has a severely depressing effect

on your immune system. Eating sweet foods of any sort interferes with the ability of your white blood cells to attack and destroy invading pathogens. The negative effect of just one glass of orange juice can linger for more than twelve hours. In addition, sugar lowers your body's ability to produce antibodies, the chemical messengers that recognize invaders and sound the alert that mobilizes your white blood cells to attack them.[1]

Another crucial immunity-related element of your diet is your intake of essential fatty acids. I've discussed the importance of these at length in the previous chapter, so here I'll just remind you that the balance of omega-3 and omega-6 fatty acids is very important for your production of the chemical messengers—hormones and eicosanoids—that tell your immune system what to do. If the balance is tipped too far in favor of the omega-6s, as it often is among people who eat a typical American diet, the pathways that create the chemical messengers won't function properly. The messages will be garbled or may not get through at all, with the result that your immune system falters and functions far below peak efficiency.

Your body also needs some support against your immune system. Let me explain that apparent contradiction. When your white blood cells—the lymphocytes—fend off an invading pathogen, as they do literally millions of times a day in a healthy person, they generate large quantities of free radicals in the process. If you're sick, your immune system will be generating free radicals at a rate that is orders of magnitude higher than when you are well. To protect yourself against the damage from the excess free radicals, you need a diet high in natural antioxidants, along with some help from antioxidant vitanutrients.

IMMUNITY AND CANCER

So far I've been discussing your immune system as if the only thing it does is protect you against illness caused by infectious agents. Your immune system, however, has an even more important function: It protects you against cancer. Your immune cells—especially the B cells and T lymphocytes, as well as the antitumor chemicals, or cytokines, such as interferon that the lymphocytes manufacture—constantly patrol your body on the lookout for your own defective cells. Defective cells are those whose genetic material has been damaged, making them potentially or actually cancerous. Cell damage of this sort happens all the time in your body, generally as a result of free radical damage. Your body's natural antioxidant defenses keep the damage down, but you must rely on continuous surveillance from a strong, efficient immune system to detect and destroy damaged cells before they begin to multiply uncontrollably.

VITANUTRIENTS FOR IMMUNITY

To maintain a strong immune defense, you need to make sure not only that you get adequate levels of protein from your diet but also that your intake of supporting vitanutrients is high. Let's look at the vitanutrients that are most important to building and maintaining your immune system. I'll discuss each one separately.*

*For detailed information, please see *Dr. Atkins' Vita-Nutrient Solution.*

Vitamin A: Infection Fighter

One of the most important immune-support vitanutrients is vitamin A. When vitamin A was discovered early in the twentieth century, it was called the anti-infective agent because it's so important for keeping your epithelial cells moist and flexible. In general, vitamin A reinforces your immune system's ability to resist infections. It's particularly helpful for protecting you against stomach "bugs" because it keeps the mucous membranes that line your intestinal tract strong and therefore impermeable to germs.

If you do contract an infection, large doses of vitamin A can do a lot to clear it up quickly. Taking 50,000 IU the moment you feel a cold coming, along with some extra vitamin C and zinc, can help keep the illness mild and short; it may even stop it in its tracks. It's also very effective for treating sinus infections.

But while vitamin A is useful for treating a temporary illness or infection, for overall immune enhancement I prefer to see my patients take mixed carotenoid supplements. Research has shown that taking 30 mg of beta-carotene daily can cause a significant improvement in immune function.[2] In particular, beta-carotene supplements improve the activity of your natural killer cells, which attack viruses and tumor cells and play an important role in preventing cancer.[3] Supplements containing mixed carotenoids—mostly beta-carotene but also other carotenes—give your immune system a boost and also give you all the other benefits of carotenoids (see Chapter 10 for more on the value of carotenoids).

The B Complex Vitamins

The complete B complex vitamins are essential for creating white blood cells. You need all of them, and you need them all in the proper ratios to do this effectively. The absence of one or the overabundance of another throws off the whole delicate balance, with a corresponding reduction in how well your body can fight off illness.

That being the case, it's hard to say that any one B vitamin is more important than the others; nevertheless, I must make a special case for vitamin B_6, also known as pyridoxine. This vitanutrient is crucial for making adequate numbers of infection-fighting T cells.[4] I strongly recommend making sure you get between 100 and 400 mg a day to keep your immunity high.

Vitamin C: The Common Cold—and Cancer

Because you're reading this book, you may already have an interest in complementary medicine. In that case, you've probably experienced for yourself how large doses of vitamin C can shorten the duration of a cold or flu. For those of you who need some convincing that this simple, inexpensive, safe vitanutrient really helps, let's look at how it works.

More than twenty different studies tell us that the primary reason vitamin C fights colds so well is that it boosts the overall function of your immune system, especially the various types of white blood cells. These cells work best when they're saturated with as much vitamin C as they can hold. Illness depletes the cells' vitamin C levels; supplements build it back up again.[5]

Cutting off respiratory illnesses quickly becomes even more important as you age, because these illnesses are more likely to turn into bronchitis or even pneumonia in older adults. Taking just 1 gram (1,000 mg) a day of extra vitamin C could cut the duration of your cold by about 20 percent. In practice, you'll get better a day or so sooner.[6]

I don't begin to have room in this book to go into the dozens and dozens of studies that show how vitamin C protects you against cancer. There are chiefly two reasons for its cancer-fighting power, however. First, it is a very robust antioxidant, which means it neutralizes free radicals before they have the chance to do the sort of damage that initiates cancer. Second, your T lymphocytes, which are one of your body's main defenses against cancer, need plenty of vitamin C to function at peak levels. In short, vitamin C is widely regarded as the most powerful anticarcinogenic nutrient known.[7] That has been borne out by epidemiological studies of eighty-eight different populations worldwide.[8] Need I say more?

Vitamin E for Excellent

One of the more interesting pieces of recent vitanutrient research is the "discovery" that vitamin E enhances immunity. This has been a well-known fact among complementary practitioners for years, but perhaps now the information will trickle down to mainstream medicine, where this sort of knowledge is badly needed. The most recent study looked at the effect of vitamin E on the immune systems of eighty-eight healthy older adults. Half took supplemental vitamin E; half took a placebo. After three months, the people taking vitamin E had measurably higher levels of T cells; after six months, their ability to produce infection-fighting antibodies was markedly higher. The best results came from the group that took 200 IU daily.[9]

If vitamin C is good for immunity and vitamin E is also good for immunity, what happens when you combine them? You get even better immunity. A recent study showed that a combined supplementation containing 1 g of vitamin C and 800 IU of vitamin E and taken for just thirty days increased several parameters of immune function in all older adults; it was especially effective for inactive older men.[10]

Let me just remind you that the results of the Third National Health and Nutrition Examination Survey (NHANES III) showed that almost 30 percent of American adults have low blood levels of vitamin E.[11] These people are setting themselves up not just for avoidable infectious disease but also for avoidable heart disease and cancer. Doses of vitamin E up to 3,200 IU daily are very safe, but you don't need to take that much. I generally recommend 1,200 IU of natural—not synthetic—vitamin E a day.

Zinc for Immune System Zing

Your body needs zinc to manufacture more than two hundred different enzymes. No zinc, no enzymes, including enzymes that are crucial to proper immune system function. Specifically, you need zinc to manufacture white blood cells and to support the activity of your neutrophils, T cells, and natural killer cells (NK cells). The NKs are the lymphocytes that kill cancer cells and fight off infections. Much of the zinc in your body is tied up in these NKs.

Other substances made with zinc play a central role in cell growth and differentiation in your body. Ironically, zinc is also important for regulating normal cell death—a sort of cellular suicide that occurs when your immune system orders defective cells to self-destruct. If the orders don't get through, the defective cells may divide uncontrollably instead. In other words, they become cancerous.

The most popular use of zinc today is in lozenges taken to fend off colds and flu. If you start using the lozenges as soon as you feel the first symptoms, you could cut down cold symptoms from an average of about a week to just four days.[12] For fighting colds, I generally recommend lozenges made with zinc gluconate with glycine. Let the lozenge dissolve slowly in your mouth; don't chew it. Adults can use a lozenge once every few hours for up to two days—don't take more than twelve lozenges in a day. Make sure each lozenge has at least 22 mg of zinc. Anything less won't do you much good.

Zinc also helps wounds heal, including the wounds of surgery. If you must have an operation, taking zinc supplements for several weeks both before and after the surgery will help you heal faster and with less chance of infection. And if you have a wound that's not healing well, it could be that you're low on zinc. Unfortunately, zinc isn't abundant in foods, and your body has a hard time absorbing what little there is. You probably need to add a zinc supplement to your daily regimen.

Zinc also acts to improve the action of your thymus gland. This is a small organ found in your neck just above your breastbone. The thymus is crucial to your health, because it makes some of the hormones that tell your immune system what to do. Your thymus gland is quite large when you're an infant, but by the time you reach your teens, it has naturally shrunk quite a bit. By the age of forty, your thymus may have shrunk so much that it can't really be found anymore. And by the time you're in your fifties, your thymus is practically nonexistent. Although a certain amount of thymus shrinking is considered normal, you certainly don't want it disappearing on you. One way to keep your thymus gland going is to make sure you get plenty of zinc. It's even possible that taking zinc supplements can revitalize your thymus and get it working again. (I'll talk more about ways to improve thymus function near the end of this chapter.)

Even though the basic daily zinc requirement is only about 15 mg for men and 12 mg for women, a distressingly large number of adults, especially older adults, are deficient.[13] A recent study of older adults in Italy found that taking 25 mg of zinc sulfate daily for three months led to an improvement in the overall status of the study participants' immune systems, based on their T-cell count. To avoid a deficiency and get the benefit of extra zinc, I suggest taking 25 mg a day.[14]

Iron-Clad Protection

Iron deficiency is one of the most common nutritional deficiencies in America. It's fairly widespread among older adults, especially those who mistakenly eat a high-carbohydrate, high-fiber, low-meat or no-meat diet. These people don't get much iron from their food, and the iron they do get is bound up in the fiber and passes through them without being absorbed. I certainly urge you to have your doctor test your blood for iron deficiency, and if a problem shows up, to treat it by adding red meat to your diet.

There is a flip side to iron, however, and that side can be dangerous in a number of ways. For one thing, excess iron in your system can lead to increased oxidation—you quite literally grow rusty. Excess iron could also feed the growth of tumor cells and harmful bacteria, as well as causing enough excess free radicals to initiate cancer-producing changes in the genetic material of your cells. And, if you're suffering from an illness or infection, especially if it's affecting your gastrointestinal tract, you should stay away from iron supplements.

In fact, I recommend that nonanemic older adults avoid extra iron from individual supplements or from multivitamin pills. But to help reduce the risk of cancer, which increases with age, there's no reason to avoid the natural iron that comes from red meat, chicken, and fish. This form, called heme iron, can't build up in your body and isn't vulnerable to oxidation.

Lest I frighten you about the consequences of iron overload, let's look at an objective study of which is better, too much or too little iron. Too little, it turns out, is much riskier than too much. According to a study of all-cause death rates of older adults, men and women with the highest blood levels of iron had 38 percent and 28 percent lower death rates, respectively.[15]

DHEA: Supplementing Your Immunity

In Chapter 12, I wrote extensively about the many virtues of DHEA. Its importance to your immune health cannot be overstated. Let me briefly review why.

The mother hormone DHEA improves your production of antibodies. It also boosts the action of the various types of white blood cells that attack and kill viruses and cancer cells, including monocytes, NK cells, and T lymphocytes. In short, taking DHEA can restore your immune system function to the level you enjoyed in your twenties and thirties, when you were probably at your healthiest.

HERBAL IMMUNE BOOSTERS

At the Atkins Center, we are very much opposed to the sort of indiscriminate antibiotic use that is widely practiced by conventional physicians. As is now widely accepted, this dangerous practice is the primary cause of the new epidemic of antibiotic-resistant pathogens. On the level of the individual patient, we find that antibiotics often cause as many problems as they solve, so whenever possible and prudent, I prefer to help the patient's own immune system do the healing. To help the immune system work its hardest, I prescribe the vitanutrients I've just discussed, along with a number of valuable herbal supplements that are proven immunity-enhancers.

First and foremost among the immunity-enhancing herbals is garlic. Rich in selenium and germanium, two trace minerals that are important for manufacturing immune cells, garlic is a broad-spectrum antimicrobial that is quite effective for destroying bacteria, including some that have become antibiotic-resistant. Taking garlic is almost certain to modify the course of any infectious disease favorably. And garlic stimulates your overall immune system, with a particularly beneficial effect on your production of natural killer cells.

Garlic is also an extremely effective antifungal. This is important because yeast infections suppress your immune system, so fighting them boosts your immunity. In fact, anyone who is prone to illness and infections should be checked for yeast infections. At the Atkins Center, we use garlic as part of our overall program for eradicating such infections. It works particularly well against *Candida albicans*, the fungus responsible for yeast overgrowths in the intestinal tract. (See Chapter 16 on detoxifying your body for more on yeast infections.)

To get the immunity-enhancing benefits of garlic, it's preferable to take 2,400 to 3,200 mg daily. That's an awful lot of garlic—enough to potentially upset your digestion, to say nothing of the powerful garlic breath you'd develop. I much prefer to have my patients take some of it as odorless, tasteless extract of dried garlic, in capsule or liquid form.

After garlic, my next favorite herbal for immunity is ginseng. Overall, ginseng is valuable as an adaptogen, an herb that helps the body adjust to stress. It is generally used as a way to improve mental and physical stamina, to the point that its value as an immunity-enhancer is sometimes overlooked. In fact, however, placebo-controlled studies tell us that taking ginseng can shorten the duration of colds and flu and may even help protect you against getting them to begin with.[16] The German Commission E, which evaluates herbs for the German government, considers ginseng a nonspecific immuno-stimulant, but there's some good evidence that ginseng works to stimulate your production of natural killer cells.[17] Recently, Danish researchers have found that ginseng enhanced the immune response to a bacterium called *Pseudomonas aeruginosa*, which causes a serious pneumonialike lung infection. The research so far is in lab rats, but there's no reason to think ginseng wouldn't also help humans infected with this dangerous organism.[18] And of course, to the extent that it relieves stress, which can be an immunity-suppressor, ginseng boosts your immune system.

Of course, ginseng is also a powerful antioxidant that has been shown to prevent lipid peroxidation. It also quenches hydroxyl, the most dangerous of the free radicals.[19]

I often suggest daily ginseng supplements to patients who are under a lot of stress or whose immunity is low. Look for a standardized supplement that contains 5 to 10 percent ginsenosides. I generally recommend 100 to 200 mg one to three times daily. The effects could take a couple of weeks or even longer to be felt. If you feel the ginseng is making you feel irritable or anxious or is disturbing your sleep, cut back on the dosage.

My final favorite herb for enhancing immunity is echinacea. This herb, made from the roots of the purple coneflower, was well-known to the Plains Indians, who introduced it to Europeans hundreds of years ago. Echinacea works by reinforcing your natural immune defenses. It's very useful not just for preventing illness, especially colds and upper respiratory infections, but also for speeding your recovery time.

During cold and flu season, I recommend taking two to three capsules a day of freeze-dried echinacea powder as a preventive. If you do get sick, taking six to eight capsules a day will help you feel better sooner.

GLUTAMINE: FUELING YOUR IMMUNE SYSTEM

The most abundant amino acid in your body is glutamine. It's also perhaps the most valuable for helping you recover from illness and injury and for keeping your immune system working at peak efficiency.

Glutamine is the primary source of energy for your immune system. You always need lots of it, but when you're sick or have an infection, your immune system goes into overdrive and requires extra fuel. If it doesn't get enough glutamine, the system will sputter along and won't be able to knock out the infectious agents effectively. You'll end up being sicker for longer.

The same is true for recovering from an injury—like a bad cut or burn—and from surgery. You need plenty of glutamine to heal the wound and nourish your immune system.[20]

Fortunately, it's easy to get all the glutamine you need by taking it in the form of an inexpensive powder. For immune support, I recommend anywhere from 5 to 20 g a day—say, one to four teaspoons, since there are about five grams in a teaspoon. If you're fighting an infectious illness or are healing from an injury or surgery, you can increase to as much as 40 g a day.

THYMUS SUPPORT

As I mentioned briefly earlier in this chapter, your thymus gland is the organ of immunity, yet it shrinks away as you get older. If your immune response needs support, it makes sense to stimulate the thymus into greater output of the hormones that the gland is responsible for making.

One possible way is with melatonin, the hormone I discussed at length in Chapter 9 in our exploration of antioxidant enzymes. This however, falls into a different category. We know that melatonin may help reverse age-related declines in your production of antibodies. Some recent research also indicates that melatonin may help reinvigorate your thymus gland, as well as your spleen and bone marrow, organs that are crucial for the production of lymphocytes.

Your thymus, spleen, and bone marrow cells all appear to have receptor sites for melatonin on them, although so far, the studies on why, and what these melatonin receptors do, have been done largely on lab rodents. The results are encouraging, however. The animals given melatonin made more antibodies and other immune system chemicals such as interleukin 2 and showed other evidence of improved immunity as well.[21] Does this mean melatonin can improve human immunity? The evidence isn't in yet, but I believe it can. Because melatonin also has other benefits as a potent antioxidant, I recommend taking it for that purpose—there may well be immune benefits as well.

Suppose you make all the dietary changes and consume all the vitanutrients I recommended in this chapter and yet you still have frequent minor illnesses. If that's the case, there's a good chance that your body is overloaded with toxins that are weakening your immune defenses. In the next chapter we'll look at techniques that can remove the toxins, restore your health, and set you squarely on the path of age defiance.

16

DETOXIFYING YOUR BODY

A legacy of the twentieth century we are very unlikely to shake off in the twenty-first is the massive, continuous exposure to toxins from our environment. There's no way to avoid them. Every day, one way or another, the typical American comes up against automobile exhaust fumes, smog, household cleaning products, tobacco smoke, paint fumes, chlorinated water, lead and such other heavy metals as cadmium, pesticides, food additives, prescription and nonprescription drugs, and many more potentially highly toxic substances.

Exposure to these substances may have serious repercussions—with as yet unknown long-term impact. For example, there are tens of thousands of industrial chemicals in use today, many of them harmful to humans at least to some degree. Each of these substances by itself is bad enough, but what happens when you're exposed to them in combination? That's a truly frightening question, and what makes it even more frightening is that nobody really knows.

Your body's waste-removal systems were never designed for the sort of toxic onslaught that most of us now experience on a daily basis. Take as one instance the chemical element cadmium. Used in many industrial processes and also found in cigarette smoke, cadmium is something humans have been exposed to only in the last couple of centuries. We don't yet have a natural detoxification pathway in our bodies that can remove the cadmium. Once it enters the body, it stays there, possibly triggering lung cancer and other diseases.

Exposure to toxins, whether naturally from the ultra-violet radiation of the sun, or unnaturally from smog and other industrial pollutants, is a major factor in aging. Why? Because toxins create free radicals—and as you certainly know at this point in this book, damage from free radicals is the underlying cause of the diseases of aging.

Your liver is the organ that is chiefly responsible for removing toxins from your body. The process is a complicated one that I won't go into in depth here. What you need to know is that the detoxifying process in the liver naturally produces a lot of free radicals. Ordinarily, those free radicals are quickly quenched by glutathione, the most abundant antioxidant enzyme in your body. When your liver is busy with extra detoxification, it needs extra glutathione, which you might not be able to make quickly enough or in large enough quantities. If you can't produce enough glutathione, the free radicals can get the upper hand in your liver and elsewhere, with serious long-term consequences.

This means that the overall formula for keeping toxins at bay is, for openers, trying to prevent the toxins from harming you in the first place, then supporting and strengthening your liver and making sure your levels of glutathione and other antioxidant enzymes stay high. In addition, there are special techniques for cleaning your liver and for ridding your body of some of the specific toxins that accelerate the aging process and make you vulnerable to degenerative diseases. In this chapter, we'll look at all these aspects of fighting toxins.

REDUCING YOUR EXPOSURE TO TOXINS

Sadly, in today's society we must simply accept that we are inevitably exposed to numerous toxins all the time. The most we can hope to do, short of moving to Alaska and living in a log cabin far from civilization, is to minimize our exposure and maximize our defenses.

To minimize your exposure, start by considering the water you drink. Your household water is probably chlorinated and fluoridated by your municipality. The chlorine and fluoride are added to kill bacteria, which means they kill all bacteria, including the beneficial bacteria in your intestines. In addition, your water may also be picking up copper and lead as it passes through metal pipes on its way to you. Even worse, it may have been contaminated along the way by dangerous pathogens, like *E. coli* or cryptosporidium, that chlorine doesn't kill. These pathogens can make you sick with severe stomach upsets. Indeed, children, the elderly, and anyone with a compromised immune system can die from the diseases prompted by these pathogens.

To protect yourself, I strongly recommend that you install household water filters on all the taps in your home. My preference is for the ceramic filters, which are reasonably priced, easy to install, and last a long time. When pure filtered water isn't available, stick to bottled water whenever possible.

The very air you breathe can also be a major source of toxins. You might think that the problem of air pollution isn't so bad if you don't live in a city that regularly has smog alerts, but that's not necessarily the case. At the Atkins Center, when patients attribute headaches, dizziness, anxiety, and "brain fog" at the office to the stress of their jobs, the first question we ask is whether they work in a sealed office building where you can't open the windows. When the answer is yes, as it often is, we've probably found the root of the problem. It isn't stress—these people are perfectly capable of doing their jobs well. It's their environment.

The sealed building typical of a suburban office park is a sinkhole for all the chemicals that can be found in today's offices. Toxic fumes from carpeting, paint, plastic furniture, copying machines, solvents, cleaning fluids, and many more substances are trapped inside the building, especially if the ventilation system is poor, as it often is. You end up breathing in these toxins, along with all the germs exhaled by your fellow workers. It's not surprising that "sick building" syndrome sometimes leads to epidemics of headaches, dizziness, rashes, and other symptoms among the workers in an office.

You can reduce the toxic level of the air around you by insisting that your work environment be properly ventilated, as federal law requires. At home and if possible at the office, use HEPA air filters, which are very good for removing toxins, particulates, and such allergens as mold spores from the air.

ARE YOU POISONING YOURSELF?

Another source of toxins in your body could very well be your own digestive system. If you can't eliminate toxins well, your overall health will suffer; if the intestinal tract accumulates toxic waste products, any health problems you do have will be exacerbated. Of even more concern are toxins created in your intestinal tract by the presence of a yeast overgrowth, also known as candidiasis. This problem has now achieved such epidemic proportions that we need to spend some time discussing its causes and treatments.

Ordinarily, your intestines contain billions of bacteria that are essential to your digestion. They are a vital part of the process that breaks down your food into nutrients you can absorb. Often, however, those beneficial bacteria get crowded out by an overgrowth of a yeastlike organism called *Candida albicans*. What causes yeast overgrowth? A host of medical and dietary abuses.

A major cause is medications—antibiotics, anti-inflammatory drugs like prednisone and ibuprofen, and birth-control pills. Poor diet plays a major role as well. The chief dietary culprit by far is excessive sugar, followed closely by insufficient fiber. In fact, in my experience, either antibiotic abuse or overconsumption of sugar—and as often as not, a combination of the two—is the most likely cause of a yeast overgrowth.

In addition, alcohol, food additives, food intolerances—especially lactose or gluten intolerance—insufficient stomach acid, and emotional stress all can trigger yeast overgrowth. Another factor in yeast overgrowth, often overlooked, is the role of untreated bacterial infections and parasites.

Approximately one in four patients at the Atkins Center is found to have a yeast overgrowth, which I believe is closely related to the larger disease picture of chronic fatigue syndrome, immune system weakness, irritable bowel syndrome, and food intolerances. The diagnosis of the condition can be reliably made by a blood test that measures for elevated IgA or IgM antibodies to candida. It can also be inferred from a variety of symptoms, especially lower intestinal gas and bloating, frequent bouts of diarrhea and constipation, decreased resistance to infection, the chronic fatigue syndrome, "brain fog," recurrent bladder infections, and thrush, a whitish plaque in the mouth and throat. Joint pain, fatigue, and depression are also common symptoms. Yeast overgrowth is also strongly associated with arthritis.[1]

When you have a yeast overgrowth, you're hosting organisms that typically produce some seventy-nine different toxins, including formaldehyde and acetaldehyde, which is exactly the same toxin you get from drinking alcohol. Acetaldehyde, in fact, is responsible for the "brain fog" that is often associated with candidiasis. The toxins from these harmful bacteria in the gut are also a possible cause of Alzheimer's disease and Parkinson's disease.[2] And yeast overgrowth in the large intestine produces massive amounts of cell-damaging free radicals, prime villains in the aging process. Only by maintaining a good balance of beneficial bacteria in your intestines can you prevent the buildup of these metabolic poisons and thus help protect against these and other diseases associated with aging.

Yeast in your intestines lives on sugar, so the first step in curing a yeast overgrowth is simply to deprive yeast of its favorite food. At the Atkins Center, we start by putting candidiasis patients on a low-carbohydrate, sugar-free diet that also eliminates all cured, fermented, or yeast-containing foods like cheese, vinegar, alcohol, and bread. Of course, patients also avoid any foods to which they have an intolerance.

We use grapefruit seed or olive leaf extracts and oil of oregano to kill off the yeast and any parasites. This very effective approach is far safer than Diflucan, the usual drug prescribed for candidiasis. But I must mention one side effect of the treatment. For the first few days, patients often feel worse instead of better. That's because the yeast cells are dying off in large numbers, which makes your intestines temporarily more toxic. I promise you that the worsened symptoms really aren't that bad and that they're worth experiencing for the improvement that follows soon after. If you feel a lot worse or if the symptoms persist, you might have to call your doctor. The results are little short of miraculous for some patients. Their health and energy are restored after years of chronic tiredness, digestive upsets, frequent illness, and poor mental function.

While you are on the antiyeast diet, you must also begin to restore a healthy balance of beneficial bacteria—also called probiotics—to your intestines. Three friendly bacteria strains are most commonly used to re-inoculate your digestive tract: bifidus, acidophilus, and lactobacillus. Most patients take capsules containing 500,000 spores of each bacteria. The doses sound huge, but remember that the bacteria themselves are microscopic—the capsules are small enough to be easily swallowed. You'll need to take one or two three times a day on an empty stomach. Treating a yeast overgrowth is a long-term project. In general, it could easily take two to four months to evict the yeast and restore a healthy balance.

Once the balance is restored, Atkins Center patients switch to the intestinal repair part of the program. We use a variety of vitanutrients to restore the integrity of your intestinal walls and build up your ability to resist unfriendly bacteria. Among the key vitanutrients are pantethine, glutamine, N-acetyl-cysteine, essential fatty acids, and gamma oryzanol (rice bran oil). We also add fiber in the form of psyllium husks, which helps your food move through your system quickly and regularly. This helps keep the yeast from gaining a foothold again. The repair process can take two to three months.

The probiotics and fiber used in the repair program are so valuable for reducing your body's toxic load, however, that I recommend them for everyone, not just as a treatment for candidiasis. By maintaining a healthy bacterial balance in the intestines, you significantly reduce your liver's workload and let it concentrate on removing the unavoidable toxins. That, in turn, helps you defy aging.

I suggest taking weekly or twice-weekly probiotic supplements of acidophilus, bifidus, and lactobacillus. One 500-mg capsule of each is enough—take them on an empty stomach. In addition, be sure that you get at least 7 to 10 grams of fiber in your diet daily. Use psyllium husks as a way to get the extra fiber if you can't get enough from the vegetables in your diet. A daily dose of one tablespoon stirred into eight ounces of plain water should do the trick.

HELPING YOUR LIVER

Your liver is the largest internal organ in your body. Every moment of every day, your liver acts like a chemical factory, producing thousands of different enzymes and other substances that affect how your body functions. Your liver is also your body's primary pathway for removing metabolic wastes and toxins from your body. It's pretty clear that keeping your liver in good working order will have a positive impact on your entire body. That means keeping it strong with vitanutrients, the right diet, and some special techniques that keep the toxins at bay.

Vitanutrients can make an enormous difference. As you remember from Chapter 9, the best way to quench the free radicals released by the liver's detoxifying process is to take in plenty of the vitanutrients your body needs to manufacture antioxidants: N-acetyl cysteine, lipoic acid, selenium, and glutathione supplements. Other vitanutrients that support your liver are also valuable, including vitamin C, vitamin E, and zinc. The zinc is particularly important for thwarting the activation of carcinogens as your liver detoxifies them.

You also need to support your liver through diet so that it functions at the optimal level and isn't overstrained. This is another area where the low-carbohydrate, high-protein diet pays off. The high-quality protein foods like red meat, poultry, seafood, and eggs enhance detoxification. A lack of protein impairs detoxification because you're not taking in enough of the amino acids, especially cysteine, that you need to make glutathione. Your liver also needs protein to manufacture bile, which is essential for absorbing fat-soluble nutrients.

Sugar in any form inhibits the production of the enzymes you need as part of the detoxification process, and this in turn will weaken liver function. To strengthen your production of detoxifying enzymes, include lots of cruciferous vegetables in your diet. These members of the cabbage family—including broccoli, kale, and Brussels sprouts—are very high in a substance called sulforaphane, which is vital for your liver's ability to convert toxins into nontoxic wastes that can then be removed from your body. And don't forget to drink plenty of pure water every day; at least two quarts—eight 8-ounce glasses—are recommended. The water flushes toxins through your system quickly and minimizes their chances to do damage.

But to really keep your liver functioning smoothly, I recommend detoxifying it every six months with a liver and gallbladder flush. This helpful procedure removes accumulated toxins and is valuable for restoring high functional capacity to these organs.

A liver flush takes three days to do, so I strongly suggest you do it over a weekend when you don't have much else scheduled. Here are the steps to follow:

1. From Monday until noon on Saturday, eat your normal diet and take your usual supplements. In addition, drink as much fresh lemon juice as your appetite permits. Dilute it with pure water to taste and sweeten it, if you wish, with stevia.

2. Eat a normal lunch at noon on Saturday.

3. Three hours later, dissolve 2 teaspoons of sodium diphosphate—you may know this under its more common name, milk of magnesia—in 1 ounce of hot water and drink. If you're like most of my patients, you'll find the taste objectionable. To get rid of it, sip some more lemon juice.

4. Repeat step 3 two hours later.

5. For your evening meal, have only fresh grapefruit, grapefruit juice, or other citrus fruits or juices.

6. At bedtime, have either 4 ounces of unrefined olive oil followed by 6 ounces of grapefruit juice, or 4 ounces of unrefined olive oil blended with 4 ounces of lemon juice. (You can buy unrefined olive oil at health food stores. Keep it refrigerated.)

7. Following step 6, go immediately to bed and lie on your right side with your right knee pulled up close to your chest. Stay that way for thirty minutes, then go to sleep.

8. The next morning, before breakfast, take 2 more teaspoons of milk of magnesia dissolved in 2 ounces of hot water. From now on, continue with your normal diet and supplements. That's it.

The liver flush has a relaxing effect on your bowels. You may notice small, light-green, irregularly shaped objects in your stool the next day. This is perfectly normal—in fact, it indicates that the liver flush has helped.

GETTING THE LEAD OUT—AS WELL AS OTHER HEAVY METALS

Lead, mercury, and cadmium are among the most common toxins that can accumulate in your body. Anyone over the age of fifty in America today is quite likely to have accumulated a toxic load of these heavy metals. Not surprisingly, that load can lead to some very serious health problems.

You've doubtless heard the expression "mad as a hatter." Well, there used to be a deadly truth behind that. The men who made hats used mercury to prepare the felt. It didn't take long for them to develop the symptoms of mercury poisoning, which include drooling, tremors, depression, and erratic behavior.

Similarly, until the use of lead paint and lead pipes was banned decades ago, housepainters and plumbers used to get lead poisoning from their work. The same reasoning was behind the ban on leaded gasoline. Exhaust fumes spread lead throughout the population and harmed the health of mechanics and gas station attendants.

The heavy metal cadmium is a by-product of many industrial processes, including zinc smelting. It can be inhaled from polluted air or ingested in contaminated food and water. If your levels of cadmium are high, you're at risk for lung cancer and kidney disease. Recent research shows that high levels of cadmium are also related to bone loss and fractures in older people, especially women. The cadmium increases your excretion of calcium, which in turn leads to thin, brittle bones that break easily.[3]

Although today your exposure to lead is less than it once was, it is almost certainly still far too high. Old lead plumbing and lead paint are still around, as is all the soil contaminated by the lead that for decades spewed out of the exhaust pipes of millions of vehicles. But mercury is still a major problem; it is widely used in many industrial applications. And of course, it comprises half the metal in the silver amalgam fillings used to fill dental cavities. If you have silver fillings, small amounts of mercury are continuously leaching into your body. I'll discuss that momentarily.

Over time, absorbing small amounts of lead can lead to anemia, neurological damage, high blood pressure, and cardiovascular disease in adults. Small children with high lead levels have impaired mental development that causes learning disabilities and behavioral problems—and lead poisoning is shamefully widespread among the poor children of America.

In one recent study, nearly 12 percent of two-year-old inner city children had mildly elevated lead levels, 4.3 percent had moderately elevated levels, and nearly 1 percent had severely elevated levels.[4] Even low levels of lead exposure can trigger behavioral changes in young children. Standard behavioral tests reveal that lead-exposed children age one to three score an average of nearly sixteen points lower than nonexposed youngsters.[5]

Your body has no mechanisms for removing lead, cadmium, and other heavy metals. Once these substances get into your system, they're there to stay—unless you remove them through chelation therapy.

CHELATION: THE DETOXIFYING KEY

Chelation (pronounced key-LAY-shun) is a chemical process that captures metal ions in your bloodstream—

including lead, iron, calcium, mercury, copper, and zinc—and binds them to an organic molecule. For all intents and purposes, the metal ion is handcuffed to the molecule and can't get away. Instead, it is carried harmlessly out of your body through the urine.

The original use of chelation, starting in the 1930s, was as a treatment for lead poisoning. Then as now, the therapy was administered intravenously. A liquid called ethylenediaminetetraacetic acid (EDTA) is slowly dripped into your blood through a thin needle inserted directly into a vein in your arm. The EDTA binds to the lead and other metals and removes them.

A typical chelation treatment takes about three hours and is completely painless (after the initial needle stick to insert the IV). To reduce a toxic load of lead, you'd probably need to have twenty or more weekly sessions. You'd also need to take zinc supplements to replenish the zinc removed by the EDTA. I also prescribe supplements of vitamin B_6. For many of my patients with elevated lead levels, chelation therapy works wonderfully well. After a dozen treatments, their levels usually drop below detectable amounts, and they feel much better.

Although chelation therapy for low-level lead exposure has long been a mainstay of complementary medicine, it is beginning to gain acceptance in the mainstream. That's probably because the evidence of chelation's usefulness keeps growing.

A recent experiment, for example, was performed on thirty-two kidney patients, all of whom had undergone long-term exposure to low levels of environmental lead and all of whom showed mildly elevated blood levels of lead. The study divided the patients into two groups. One group received IV chelation therapy with EDTA; the other did not. The researchers reported that chelation slowed the progression of renal insufficiency, or kidney failure, in the patients and actually improved their kidney function by an average of 8.5 percent.[6]

Another study of low-level lead poisoning is the Treatment of Lead-exposed Children trial, the TLC trial. This study uses an oral chelation agent called succimer to reduce lead levels in toddlers. Succimer is an "orphan" drug also known as Chemet that is quite expensive; special permission from the FDA is required for its use. It's highly effective, and it's not at all the same thing as the oral chelation products that are peddled by some promoters as being just as good as IV chelation for removing toxins from the body. Oral chelation may indeed offer some help for low-level toxic buildup, but in my experience it is not as effective as IV chelation.

BYPASSING BYPASS SURGERY WITH CHELATION

Overall, chelation therapy is a valuable part of your age-defying program. By removing accumulated heavy metals from your body, you not only remove their harmful effects but also reduce the amount of free radicals they produce. At the Atkins Center, however, we get our most spectacular chelation results from patients with heart disease.

We have treated thousands of patients whose conventional doctors warned them that only an immediate angioplasty or heart bypass surgery would save their lives. These patients come to us desperately seeking an alternative to these dangerous procedures, knowing that in fact many bypass patients get worse, not better after the surgery. They find the alternative they need in IV chelation therapy, and they also save thousands of dollars. Chelation is far less expensive, and of course far safer, than open-heart surgery or angioplasty.

How exactly does chelation help heart disease? In several ways. Unlike bypass surgery or angioplasty, which deal with just a few of the hundreds of arteries in your body, chelation therapy simultaneously increases blood flow in all your major blood vessels, including the ones that nourish the heart, kidneys, brain, and other organs. This happens in part because the EDTA removes some of the calcium found in artery-clogging plaque. The reduction in calcium can reduce or may even eliminate the plaque. Even when plaque isn't reduced or removed, the reduction in calcium makes the artery more flexible.

Chelation also lowers the level of calcium in your blood, which then stimulates your body to release parathyroid hormone, which in turn stimulates your body to remove calcium from places it doesn't belong—like your arteries—and put it where it does belong—like your bones. In that way, EDTA causes a recalcification of osteoporotic bones.[7] And, by removing lead, mercury, cadmium, and other accumulated heavy metals, chelation removes another cause of heart damage.

EDTA offers heart patients a number of other benefits. One of the most valuable is stimulating the enlargement of small blood vessels near blocked arteries. These small vessels create collateral circulation around the blockage—your body's own natural bypass. EDTA is also a powerful antioxidant that can help reduce LDL cholesterol oxidation.[8] Also very helpful for heart patients is EDTA's anticoagulant qualities, which reduce platelet "stickiness" and help prevent blood clots that can cause a heart attack.[9]

Given all the benefits of chelation therapy, it's puzzling that insurance companies and Medicare refuse to pay for it. These organizations will cheerfully pay $50,000 for you to have bypass surgery, but they won't give you a penny toward the few thousand dollars that buy a complete course of chelation therapy.

In fact, conventional physicians often scoff at chelation. Some have tried to ban it as a treatment. The issue regularly comes up before state medical regulatory boards, but despite what your doctor may tell you, chelation is readily available and perfectly legal just about everywhere in the United States. To find a trained physician who can help you with chelation, check with the American College for Advancement in Medicine (ACAM) at (800) 532-3688.

MERCURY DETOXIFICATION

Mercury, as we've seen, is a highly toxic heavy metal that is extremely dangerous to your health. Mercury exposure is a significant cause of such autoimmune diseases as multiple sclerosis, psoriasis, and chronic fatigue syndrome. It's a significant contributor to cancer and heart disease. Anyone who lives in our modern industrial society has been exposed to considerable amounts of mercury over his or her lifetime: it's widely used in many industrial processes and in a range of commonly used chemicals. At one time it was even used in interior housepaint as a way to prevent mildew, a use that was banned several decades ago. There's a very good chance that as you read this book, you are being slowly poisoned by mercury. How? From the silver amalgam fillings in your teeth.

Although the dental establishment steadfastly denies it, silver amalgam, a common material widely used as an inexpensive method to fill the holes in your teeth left by cavities and root canal procedures, consists of only about 25 percent silver. Half the amalgam is mercury;

the rest is a mixture of other metals, including tin, zinc, and copper.

According to the World Health Organization, just one silver amalgam filling in your mouth can release 3 to 17 micrograms of mercury a day.[10] Every time you brush your teeth or chew on something, your fillings are releasing tiny amounts of mercury into your body. This is especially true of old fillings, which can corrode over time. Remember, your body has no natural metabolic pathway to remove that mercury. It just accumulates in your body.

In Germany, mercury amalgam fillings have been banned since 1992. Here in the United States we are far less enlightened, although there are some holistic dentists who are aware of the issue and refuse to use silver amalgam.

Right now, the best alternative to a silver amalgam is a polymer ceramic. This material is very hard and durable and contains no metals. It's also much more natural-looking than silver amalgam. But ceramic fillings are more expensive than standard amalgam fillings, so should you be fortunate enough to have dental insurance, you'll find that your insurer almost certainly won't pay for the extra cost.

Providing you locate a dentist experienced in the safe removal of silver amalgam fillings, I urge you to replace all of yours with ceramic fillings and pay every penny of the cost yourself if necessary. The long-term expense of chronic illness and a shortened life span from the effects of mercury will cost you far more than the fillings. You may have to search a bit to find a holistic dentist who will be willing to work with you. The ADA officially says that removing serviceable silver amalgam fillings from a patient is unethical, and dentists who do so risk having their licenses revoked. To find a holistic dentist who can help you, contact the Environmental Dental Association at (800) 388-8124.

Sometimes a tooth is so decayed or damaged that the root is affected. To solve the problem, dentists have traditionally performed root canal surgery to remove the infected material and fill the resulting large hole in the tooth with silver amalgam. There's a big problem with this common procedure: It can leave a residual bacterial infection at the base of the tooth. Toxins from the infection seep into your body and can stimulate chronic degenerative diseases. Many of our multiple sclerosis patients at the Atkins Center tell us that their symptoms began soon after they had root canal work involving both infection and silver amalgam fillings. I, along with many other complementary physicians who treat MS, feel that this strong correlation is no coincidence. As part of our treatment protocols for MS, we recommend removing all teeth with root canals and replacing all silver amalgam fillings.

Today's dentists are as dedicated to saving a tooth as physicians are to saving a life. Unfortunately, the two goals aren't always compatible. Having a root canal procedure could jeopardize your health and shorten your life. If at all possible, take every step you can to avoid this sort of dental surgery. Good dental hygiene will help you avoid the problem. As a last-resort alternative to a root canal, you may have to have the affected tooth removed instead. Likewise, if you have a degenerative disease like chronic fatigue syndrome, removing teeth with root canals and replacing all silver amalgam fillings— that is, removing a source of infection and of harmful mercury—could help restore your health.

The only way to remove the accumulated mercury from your system is to take a course of mercury chelation therapy—there is no other way. The chelating agents we use are called DMPS, which is given by vein, or the oral agent DMSA, of which most patients need to take one 500-mg capsule a day on 15 to 30 occasions.

MERCURY AND YOUR HEART

Cardiologists such as myself, who are aware of environmental toxins, have long known that people with high mercury levels are more likely to suffer heart failure. This has been confirmed by many studies. The most recent one looked at patients with idiopathic dilated cardiomyopathy, a common form of heart failure, and saw that the patients typically have extremely high levels of trace elements, particularly mercury and antimony. "Extremely high" is putting it mildly: Compared to patients with heart ailments due to a known cause, the idiopathic heart failure patients had mercury levels that were an astonishing 22,000 times higher.[11]

Heart patients at the Atkins Center are routinely tested for their mercury levels. Just as routinely, we find that the levels are high and must be brought down with chelation therapy. We usually treat these patients intravenously with DMPS and administer it at the same time as chelation with EDTA. To remove mercury from the body this way, we give a course of chelation treatments, each lasting about three hours.

With the toxins out of your body, with the right high-protein, low-carbohydrate diet fueling it, and with vitanutrients boosting your immunity and vigor, there's still something else you can do to turn your body into an antiaging machine: Exercise!

17

EXERCISE!

There's one piece of advice I give to virtually every one of my patients, no matter how old: Exercise. There's not a one of them who can't benefit from exercising regularly to the maximum possible for that individual. That doesn't necessarily mean that all my patients turn into marathon runners and weekend warriors, or that you will, or even that you should. What it does mean is that you'll look better, feel better, and stay healthier when you exercise. Mentally and physically, exercise makes you stronger and more resilient.

EXERCISE FOR A HEALTHY HEART

Just consider the results of a recent review of dozens of studies on the impact of physical activity on cardiovascular health. Without question, the researchers concluded, regular physical activity provides a wide range of heart-healthy benefits, including lower blood pressure, a drop in cholesterol levels, and a lower risk of dangerous blood clots. The activity doesn't have to be particularly strenuous or prolonged to be effective. Just walking once around the block each day is enough to provide some benefit.[1] Walking more would be better, of course. How much better? According to a recent study of older men in Hawaii, your risk of coronary heart disease decreases 15 percent for every half mile of walking per day.[2]

Earlier studies have shown that of all the factors most likely to lead to heart disease, inactivity is at the top of the list, far above all the usual indicators like high cholesterol.[3] Need I say more? Yes, because exercise does far more for you than just protecting your heart. It actually acts as a catalyst for all the health-enhancing, age-defying advice in this book. Put it this way: Without exercise, you'll still benefit from the advice in this book, but with exercise, you'll benefit even more.

THE BENEFITS OF EXERCISE

Age defiance, disease prevention, weight loss, and a sense of well-being are among the many benefits of regular exercise.

To defy age, it is of course crucial to keep your blood sugar levels steady and under control. Exercise is just as important as diet for accomplishing this goal. At the Atkins Center, thousands of patients with impaired glucose tolerance have successfully reversed the process and prolonged their lives through the combination of exercise and diet. That success is confirmed by studies so numerous that I won't go into them all here; suffice it to say that the studies prove that exercise can prevent, slow, or reverse reduced glucose tolerance and insulin sensitivity as you age, and even reverse diabetes if you already have it.

And the converse is equally true, as numerous other studies confirm: Not exercising means you're more likely to develop impaired glucose tolerance or diabetes, even if you're not overweight, although being overweight is certainly a contributing factor. A recent study proves this point very powerfully. It tracked more than 8,600 men over age thirty through a six-year period during which 149 men in the study developed diabetes. It didn't surprise me that the diabetes diagnoses were almost entirely among the men who were the least active. Inactive men had nearly four times the risk of developing diabetes as did the physically active men.[4]

My theory is that a vicious cycle helps explain this. Inactivity leads to weight gain, which in turn leads to diabetes, which further contributes to weight gain, which makes you feel sluggish and less interested in being physically active, and so on.

For those of you who need to lose weight, regular exercise will help speed the process along. I particularly recommend it for people who have a high metabolic resistance to weight loss. Even though walking a mile burns only a hundred calories, a prolonged exercise program often proves to be the essential that tips the balance in hard-core unable-to-lose-on-a-strict-diet people. Those of you whose weight loss is simply plateauing will find that exercise will also get you over the logjam more quickly. Best of all, the experience of seeing your fat turn into muscle, and of knowing that you are capable of many more physical achievements, is such a mood-lifter that your all-around well-being will reach new heights.

One more disease-fighting benefit: An active lifestyle is also linked with a reduced risk of cancer, as has been demonstrated in regard to colon cancer in men and breast cancer in women.[5]

THE BIGGER PICTURE

Exercise is the key factor in preventing disability as you age. It's also a key factor in overall longevity. Let's look at some statistics to prove my point.

Overall, a sixty-five-year-old man with no disabilities in the United States today has only a 26 percent chance of living to age eighty and remaining disability-free. For a woman, the probability of living to age eighty-five and remaining disability-free is only 18 percent. What does that disability-free minority do to get and stay that way? They exercise.

People who exercise regularly have a lower risk of becoming disabled later in life than those who don't exercise. And the people with the highest level of physical activity are nearly twice as likely to be disability-free as the most sedentary.[6]

What the numbers show most starkly is that disability is not an inevitable part of aging. It can easily be defied by moderate physical activity, starting now.

Physical activity can also extend your life expectancy. Among nonsmokers at age sixty-five, moderate physical activity is associated with 14.4 years of continuing life expectancy in men and 16.2 years in women. In other words, a man who exercises moderately and doesn't smoke is likely to live to be just over seventy-nine years old. That's a gain of seven years over the average life expectancy of seventy-two years for a man.

The benefits of physical activity hold true even for smokers. Male smokers who exercise moderately gain 10.5 years of extra life expectancy; women gain 12.6 years.[7] What better reason could there be to start your age-defying exercise program today?

EXERCISING YOUR OPTIONS

Despite the perfectly obvious benefits of exercising, some 30 percent of the American population doesn't exercise at all. Whether they realize it or not, these couch potatoes have opted for a shortened life span marred at the end by years of expensive, painful disability.

What will you opt for? Will you choose to exercise and defy age, or remain inactive and court disability and premature death? It's a simple choice, really, and yet I find many of my patients have trouble making the commitment to exercise. I've heard every excuse in the book, and although I'm certainly guilty of some of them myself, none of them are valid.

Patients tell me all the time that they just don't have time to exercise. I don't buy that one at all. If the average American can find time to watch six hours of mindless television a day, he or she can find time for half an hour of exercise. If you can't bear to miss a minute of TV time, ride an exercise bike or do stretching exercises and calisthenics while you watch.

Another big excuse I hear is being too old to exercise. This is just as nonsensical as the lack of time excuse. It's never too late to start an exercise program. In one study, a group of frail, nonagenarian men living in a nursing home did weight training! In just eight weeks they showed remarkable increases in muscle strength—up to 175 percent. More important, their walking speed and coordination improved by nearly 50 percent, making them much less likely to have a fall.[8] Several other studies since then have shown similar results, with elderly study participants improving walking speed and overall strength and improving measures of physical disability.[9]

"Exercise is so boring," some of my patients say. "Maybe so," is my reply, "but it's a lot less boring than living in a nursing home." Find a form of exercise you enjoy and do it regularly. Golf, tennis, walking, hiking, biking, dancing, swimming—all will roll back the clock. And even such constructive activities as gardening, housework, and home repairs can be done in such a way that they are meaningful sources of exercise.

Of all the excuses I hear, the lest convincing of all is that you are too out of shape to exercise. That's exactly what we're going to remedy!

AEROBICS AND WEIGHT TRAINING

Aerobics and weight training are the buzzwords of exercise workouts, and indeed, both are important.

Aerobic exercises are any exercises that comfortably raise your body's oxygen requirements and pulse rate and keep the rate constant for a meaningful period of time. For many of you, half an hour of brisk walking will do it; for others, it will take more to get the benefit. Low-impact jogging, bicycling, and aerobic workouts are all appropriate, providing they are not so vigorous that they stress your immune reserves or lead to injury.

Weight training, also known as resistance training, is done primarily to build up stronger muscles. It can also be moderately aerobic, especially when done with lighter weights. As mentioned earlier, research has shown that even frail, elderly people can benefit from weight training. But to avoid injury when you're first getting started with weights, I suggest working with a trainer to learn the basics.

WALKING TO BETTER HEALTH

So which exercise is best for you? Whichever one you'll enjoy enough to do regularly! If cornered, however, the form of exercise I recommend most, especially if you're just starting an exercise program, is walking. If a couch potato starts by simply taking a short walk every day, or even every other day, he or she will show dramatic improvements in a very short time.

It matters little how far or how fast you go or how old you are. In a recent study from Japan, for example, middle-aged men who walked just ten to twenty minutes a day, five days a week, reduced their risk of hypertension by 12 percent and lost weight.[10]

Another recent study, more to the point, followed nearly 3,000 American men age seventy-one to ninety-three for four years. During that time, 109 of the men were diagnosed with coronary artery disease. What's interesting is the breakdown. The men who walked 1.5 miles a day or more had a 2.5 percent risk of heart disease. The men who walked less than a quarter of a mile a day had double the risk, or a 5 percent chance of heart disease.[11] In other words, by spending half an hour taking a relaxing walk, these older men cut their risk of heart disease in half, to say nothing of the other benefits they reaped.

The benefits of walking might be even more dramatic for women. According to a recent study of participants in the ongoing Nurses' Health Study, fully one-third of heart attacks in women of any age could be prevented by three hours of brisk walking spread across a week— brisk walking means twenty minutes per mile. A woman who walks briskly for five or more hours a week cuts her heart attack risk in half. The benefit applies to all women, even sedentary ones who take up walking later in life. There's no real reason to think that what works for women won't also work for men.[12]

What other benefits does walking give you? Well, aside from the health advantages I've already discussed for any sort of exercise, walking seems to improve your mental fitness. In particular, a recent study shows that walking improves what are known as the executive control functions: your ability to plan, coordinate, and focus on information. The study compared two groups of previously sedentary older adults. One group walked for forty-five minutes three times a week. The other group did stretching and toning exercises for an hour three times a week. When the two groups were given a battery of psychological tests after six months, the walkers did much better. What seems to have made the difference is the increased flow of blood to the brain that came with walking.[13]

Walking has several other benefits to commend it. It is a weight-bearing exercise, which means it can help prevent or slow osteoporosis. It is also far gentler on your body than jogging or running and is unlikely to injure you. Unlike more strenuous forms of exercise, walking does not have a negative effect on your immune system. Jogging for just half an hour every day can significantly reduce the number of immune cells in your blood, but walking half an hour a day will have no effect on your immunity—except that it may well give it a boost.[14]

One of the best things about walking is that it requires no special equipment beyond a comfortable pair of shoes. You also don't need any special training—you've been walking all your life. And it's free—no gym fees, no fancy equipment, no instructors.

Your age-defying goal is to take a brisk, half-hour walk at least three times a week, and preferably every day. The time you spend walking is more important than the distance you cover. If you haven't walked more than a couple of blocks in years, ease into it by walking as quickly as is comfortable for just ten minutes. Gradually work up to half an hour, keeping the pace at whatever is comfortable for you. You'll be amazed at how quickly you get up to half an hour and at how much better you feel, both physically and mentally. In fact, you may feel so good that you decide to walk longer or more frequently, which in turn will make you feel even better. Talk about a win-win situation!

As you walk, be aware of your posture. We all have a natural tendency as we get older to stoop forward a bit, a tendency that can be quite pronounced in the elderly. You need to counteract the tendency before it happens. The farther forward you stoop, the more likely you are to have a fall that could break a bone.

Check your posture by standing naturally up against a wall and seeing how much of you touches it. If the back of your head doesn't touch the wall, you'll need to take some corrective steps. Before leaving the wall, try to stand so that your head *does* touch the wall. You'll find it works better if you pull your abdomen in, thrust your hips forward and try to elevate your chest away from your pelvis. This is the very posture you should strive for when walking.

As you walk, hold your chin up. Once your head is balanced more naturally over your shoulders, the rest of your posture will straighten up as well. By constantly reminding yourself to keep your head back, you'll overcome your forward stoop.

The recommendation to go walking holds true for those with arthritis or some other condition that impairs your mobility; at least, walk as much as you can. For these patients, I also recommend water exercises under the supervision of a trained physical or exercise therapist. Many local Ys and community pools offer inexpensive water exercise classes.

STRETCHING THE TRUTH

As great an age-defier as walking is, it is tied for first place in my mind with another activity that is invaluable and not at all strenuous—stretching.

I don't think I have to remind you that stiffness and progressive inflexibility of the spine and other joints are well-known accompaniments to aging. The technique of loosening up these joints by putting the tight muscles around them "on the stretch" is a dramatically effective correction for this problem.

There are probably over a hundred different stretching exercises that can benefit your different muscle groups. It's not within the scope of this book to provide the details—you can get them from the many good books on the topic or from an exercise instructor at your local Y or health club. I merely want to point out that stretches provide an invaluable protection against the musculo-skeletal problems associated with advancing years.

WHEN MORE IS LESS

If mild exercise is good and moderate exercise is better, does that make heavy exercise the best? Precisely the opposite. Aside from increasing the chances of an injury, heavy exercise stimulates you to produce an over-abundance of free radicals, has a detrimental effect on your immune system, and makes you release more of the damaging stress hormone cortisol. That's why I don't recommend running or jogging as exercise. Swimming, walking, yoga, and other slower, gentler activities—even housework—when done regularly have just as beneficial an effect on your body without all the extra wear and tear.

And anyone who thinks he or she is achieving immortality the Ornish way by running forty miles a week and eating a very low-fat diet is in for a surprise. A recent study showed that when high-mileage runners ate a diet in which only 17 percent of the calories came from fat, their levels of infection-fighting white blood cells and cytokines plummeted, while their levels of cortisol and inflammation-producing prostaglandins increased. When the runners went to a high-fat diet with 41 percent of the calories from fat, their levels returned to normal, and their level of natural killer cells, which attack viruses and tumor cells, doubled.[15] Scientific studies don't usually discuss how the subjects actually feel, but I'm sure in this case that the subjects felt a lot better in general when they were eating the high-fat diet. I'm also sure they were a lot less likely to get sick with the sort of minor ailments, like colds and infections, that dog many serious athletes who follow fat-restricted diets.

GETTING STARTED

If you're over age forty-five, before you undertake any exercise program more strenuous than brisk walking, see your doctor and get yourself examined for any cardio-vascular problems.

To avoid injuries, always do some stretching and limbering exercises before you get into the more active part of your exercise routine. If you're just beginning an exercise program, start slowly. Forget that old saying, "No pain, no gain." At first, do a little bit less than you think you can, not a little bit more. Gradually build up to a level that leaves you feeling energized and refreshed, not exhausted and sore. Over the first few weeks, you'll be amazed at how quickly you get into better shape. After that, your progress may be a bit slower. Set realistic goals for yourself and remember that you're not training for the Olympics.

When you exercise, there should be a normal elevation of your pulse rate. If you feel dizzy, have chest pains, or feel very short of breath, STOP. Check things out with your physician before you exercise to that level again. Avoid exercising outdoors in extremely hot or cold weather. When the weather is against you, try walking at your local shopping mall. You'll find you're not alone: Squads of retirees and younger folk on their way to work may be taking advantage of the climate-sheltered empty walkways to stride briskly to better health and fitness.

THE TWENTY-EIGHT-DAY GET-STARTED EXERCISING PLAN

Prior to initiating any course of exercise, you should consult with your physician. Always warm up before beginning (five minutes of gentle stretching or other slow, focused movement may do it), and cool down at the end of the exercise (stretching/walking at a slow pace).

Week 1: Walk 10 to 15 minutes at a slow to moderate pace (2½ to 3 miles per hour), one to two times a week.

Week 2: Increase rate to a steady moderate pace (3

miles per hour) and the time to 15 to 20 minutes, two times a week.

Week 3: Add 5 to 10 minutes for a walk for 20 to 25 minutes (3 to 3½ miles per hour) two to three times a week. Pump your arms while walking to increase cardiovascular benefit.

Week 4: Walk for 30 to 35 minutes three times a week, while maintaining a brisk pace (3½ to 4 miles per hour).

Now that you've started, keep it up, and aim for a daily dose of exercise.

If walking is not an option for you, try swimming, biking, low-impact aerobic exercise, or yoga. You will need to vary your routine so that it does not become boring, so change the course of your walk and/or try the above exercise options.

If you experience pain or have trouble breathing, stop exercising and consult your physician.

Whatever exercise you do should be done regularly. You'll find that it soon becomes a very pleasant routine and an essential part of your life. In fact, it can be habit-forming—if not downright addictive. Nothing could be better for you than this particular addiction. It will help ensure a sound body for life—reason enough to look now at ways to keep a sound mind in that sound body for life.

18

BOOSTING YOUR BRAIN POWER

Whenever patients ask me about one of their aging relatives, I usually start by asking, "What do you think of his or her short-term memory?" That symptom may well be the most consistent shortcoming found in people suffering what we think of as the effects of aging.

When loss of short-term memory is a progressive disorder, it becomes one of the primary symptoms of Alzheimer's disease, the victims of which are eventually unable to recognize their loved ones or even feed themselves. But more often, the decline in short-term memory remains just a nuisance, not an illness. Medically speaking, it goes by the name "age-related memory loss."

The term suggests that some loss of the ability to recall the events of the previous day or the names of familiar people is an unavoidable fact of growing older. It is not.

There are many nutrients that make a difference in maintaining, or even improving, not only your memory but all aspects of your brain power—too many nutrients for age-related memory loss to be inevitable. It's just a matter of deciding which particular nutrients are the best for you.

These nutrients are safe and quite effective. College students can use them to ace their exams, business executives can use them to rise to the top of the corporate ladder, and all of us can use them to keep our brain function high so we remain in our mental prime.

We'll look at the major brain-boosting vitanutrients in some detail in this chapter: what they are, what they do, how much to take if you think you can benefit from their use. First, however, it's important to understand how it is that these particular vitanutrients can make a difference to memory, mental acuity, and overall brain power.

WHY YOU NEED TO PROTECT YOUR BRAIN

Everything you do to protect your body from aging applies even more to your brain. That's because your brain is much more vulnerable than the rest of your body to the effects of free radicals and reduced blood flow. Why is your brain so unprotected? To answer that question, I'll touch on just a few key points of brain physiology.

Your brain consists of trillions of nerve cells, or neurons, all packed very closely together into an organ that weighs only about three pounds. All those cells communicate with each other and with the rest of your body through complex chemical messengers called neurotransmitters.

Even though your brain takes up only about 2 percent of your body mass, it demands more than 25 percent of your body's basic fuels, in the form of glucose or ketones, to run at peak efficiency.

Since glucose is the most widely examined and documented of the fuels, I'll describe how the brain uses it. First of all, brain cells are very sensitive to levels of glucose: Too little or too much can cause damage, even death. Unlike many other substances in your bloodstream, glucose passes easily through the blood-brain barrier. And unlike the cells everywhere else in your body, brain cells don't need insulin to carry the glucose into them.

If your brain cells don't need insulin, how does your body control how much glucose gets in? Through a very complex system of hormones and feedback loops, all designed to keep your blood glucose stable on the other side of the blood-brain barrier. In other words, if your body's blood sugar stays stable, your brain's will as well. The reverse is also true. If your body's blood sugar zooms up and down, or stays consistently too high, the instability will take a toll on your brain as well as on the rest of your body.

Too much glucose entering your brain has exactly the same effect as too much glucose anywhere else in your body. It causes AGEs—the advanced glycation end-products discussed in Chapter 5—as well as atherosclerosis, reduced oxygen flow, and, of course, major free radical damage. And AGEs, we've learned, contribute to the beta-amyloid plaques that are found in the brains of Alzheimer's patients.[1]

What if your brain doesn't get enough glucose? Then the hormonal feedback loop calls on a range of other substances to raise the glucose level, with varying effects.

First, it calls on glucagon. If that doesn't work—and in people with unstable blood sugar, it doesn't—the next step is to call on cortisol, the stress hormone. Your body is designed to use cortisol only when there's a sudden urgent need to raise your blood sugar—for example, when you're in a threatening situation. If unstable blood sugar frequently forces your body to fall back on cortisol, the long-term effects on your brain are quite damaging.

To be bluntly specific, cortisol kills brain cells in your hippocampus, the part of your brain that tells the rest of your brain to start the hormonal cascades. Your hippocampus is also involved in the process that turns short-term memory into long-term memory. Clearly, damage to your hippocampus cells is something you want to avoid.

A third glucose-elevating hormone is adrenaline, and its effects are highly noticeable. The adrenalinelike neurotransmitters create an emotional response of anxiety or fear characterized by rapid heartbeat, dry mouth, and sweaty palms. This explains why panic attacks and bouts of heart rhythm irregularities are triggered by falling blood sugar. Even worse, such physical and emotional stress will cause further cortisol elevations. Clearly, maintaining stable blood sugar is essential for protecting your brain.

In addition to requiring the fuel of glucose, of course, your brain needs oxygen. In fact, the brain is a glutton for oxygen, taking more than 20 percent of the blood's total supply. If the vessels that carry blood to and from your brain become stiff or partially blocked, the oxygen flow to your brain is reduced, as is the flow of everything else your brain needs. Poor cerebral circulation causes slow, steady loss of brain function: poor memory, confusion, inability to concentrate, fatigue, depression, anxiety. It also sharply increases your chance of a major stroke.

And by now you can guess that when the overall blood flow to your brain is reduced, the damage caused by lack of oxygen, glucose, and antioxidants lets free radicals get the upper hand. Free radical damage anywhere in your body is bad. In your brain, it can be devastating. Because your brain has so many cells in it, and because the membranes of those cells have such high concentrations of the fatty substances called lipids, your brain is very vulnerable to free radical damage from lipid peroxidation.

Over the long term, anything that causes free radical damage reduces brain function. Conversely, over the long term, anything that reduces free radical damage preserves brain function.

HOW TO HELP YOUR BRAIN

You may have heard the folk wisdom that you lose a hundred thousand brain cells every day as you age. It is true that some of your neurons naturally die as you get older, but in healthy aging, neuron loss is actually fairly minimal—and it happens in only some areas of the brain. It's also not true that you never grow any new neurons. In fact, even elderly people create hundreds of new neurons every day. When a neuron does die, other neurons in the area pick up the slack and create new connections with other brain cells. Have you ever seen an experienced older athlete beat the pants off a younger, faster, stronger athlete? In the same way as experience can compensate for reduced strength and speed, so your brain can compensate for the loss of neurons as you get older.

The process works a lot better, of course, if you give your brain a little help. As with your body, that help should consist of diet and exercise.

BRAIN FOOD, BRAIN WORKOUT

By diet I mean the same low-carbohydrate, high-antioxidant, high-fat diet that helps the rest of your body.

Where the brain is concerned, however, I emphasize the high fat part of the diet. The reason? Without enough essential fatty acids—the fats you must get from your food—your brain simply won't work right (check back to Chapter 14 for more on essential fatty acids).

The low-fat diet the medical establishment insists is good for you is more likely eventually to slow your brain down than to keep it going strong. New studies support this, including one showing that the typical high-fat Western diet is linked to a lower risk of poststroke dementia. The study looked at a group of older Japanese-American men who had had strokes. The men who preferred a Western-style diet to the traditional low-fat Japanese diet were about half as likely to develop stroke-related dementia, an aftermath of stroke in which the brain does not fully recover. The researchers believe that the high fat intake of the Western diet acts as a stabilizer to the small arteries in the brain.[2]

Exercise, too, is essential for keeping the brain strong and limber—the same thing it does for the body. Several studies show, for instance, that people with higher levels of education are less likely to develop Alzheimer's disease as they age.[3] The reason may well be that these people continue to stay mentally active through their work and through their leisure. You don't need a Ph.D. to read, listen to music, do crossword puzzles, or enjoy a hobby. Staying engaged and active in your community and social life also helps keep your mind sharp. The evidence is clear that socializing with family and friends and participating in group activities reduce stress levels— and therefore brain-damaging cortisol levels.[4] Anything that keeps your brain engaged will do a lot to keep it healthy.

BRAIN VITANUTRIENTS

Every few months, a new patient comes to see me at the Atkins Center complaining of forgetfulness. Suddenly, he or she just can't remember minor things that used to come easily to mind—the name of the boss's spouse, the title of a book, who was President your senior year in college. After some simple memory tests and a quick exam, I'm almost always able to give these patients good news. All they're experiencing is normal, age-related changes in their short-term memory.

If you're over forty-five, you're likely to be experiencing the same thing. Do you now have to spend the rest of your life forgetting phone numbers? No. You're fortunate to live in a time when research into brain vitanutrients is moving along very rapidly. The vitanutrients I'm about to discuss are excellent for maintaining and improving total mental function, including short-term memory.

GINKGO BILOBA

It was back in Chapter 11, talking about antioxidant vitanutrients, that I touched briefly on ginkgo biloba. Here I'll focus on the use of ginkgo to maintain and improve your mental acuity, an area in which I consider ginkgo supreme among all the brain-boosting vitanutrients.

We know from more than forty research studies that the active ingredients in ginkgo biloba are very effective for increasing blood flow to the brain. Better blood flow means better memory and more alertness overall; it can also reduce or even eliminate such symptoms as confusion, disorientation, and agitation. Of course, better blood flow also means less likelihood of a stroke. Ginkgo provides additional stroke protection by making your platelets less sticky, therefore less likely to clot, and therefore less likely to block the blood flow to your brain.

Taking ginkgo biloba on a regular basis improves your production of neurotransmitters. Typically, neurotransmitters last for only the fraction of a second it takes to transmit a message from one brain cell to another. After that, special enzymes break them down and recycle them. The neurotransmitter production and recycling processes slow down with age, leading to slower message transmission and accumulated "garbage" in the gap between neurons. Ginkgo helps you manufacture, clear away, and reuse more of these essential messenger chemicals more efficiently. It also makes the neurons themselves more sensitive to the messages they send and receive; with the neurotransmitter serotonin, for example, it seems to protect the receptor cells that respond to these neurotransmitters.

This could be why ginkgo can help slow, perhaps stop, or even reverse some of the brain damage from Alzheimer's disease.[5] In fact, in Germany and some other countries, ginkgo is an approved Alzheimer's treatment. Several recent studies in the United States have shown that taking ginkgo can stabilize and even improve Alzheimer's-type dementia for up to a year. In the studies, the patients taking ginkgo had stable or improved cognitive function. They did as well as other patients taking more expensive prescription drugs, without the side effects, and they did markedly better than patients who took only a placebo.[6]

Always choose a ginkgo supplement in tablet form

that has been standardized to 24 percent ginkgo flavonoids and 6 percent terpenes. For adults over forty, I
recommend taking at least one 60-mg tablet three times
a day for a total of 180 mg. For adults over sixty, or if
you're experiencing short-term memory loss, increase
the dose to two or even three 60-mg tablets three times
a day, for a total of 360 to 540 mg. Even doses much
larger than this are safe. Ginkgo has no known toxicity
or side effects, and it has no known interactions with
other drugs or nutrients.

When you take ginkgo biloba to improve general alertness and mental acuity, the effect is felt almost immediately. But ginkgo isn't a stimulant; it won't keep
you up at night or make you jittery.

For improving short-term memory, however, and this
is mostly why I recommend ginkgo, you'll need to take
ginkgo for at least a couple of weeks before you start
noticing a change for the better. The change happens
gradually, but almost all my patients experience significant short-term memory improvement within three
months.

PHOSPHATIDYL SERINE (PS)

If there were a safe, inexpensive dietary supplement that
could turn back a decade's worth of mental decline,
would you take it? You bet you would. Well, there is
such a supplement: phosphatidyl serine (PS). This one is
providing especially exciting results, and I find it every
bit as effective as ginkgo and complementary to it.

Phosphatidyl serine is a phospholipid—a large fatty
molecule that serves as a building block of cell membranes. The cell membranes of your brain cells are particularly rich in PS, because PS plays an important role

in both releasing neurotransmitters and increasing the number of neurotransmitter receptor sites on each cell. That gives your brain more circuits with which to communicate. As you age, though, your brain cells start to make less and less PS, to the point where eventually your cognitive ability is impaired. The deterioration will happen faster if you're also low on the building blocks for manufacturing PS in your body: folic acid, vitamin B_{12}, and essential fatty acids, particularly the omega-3 oils.

Taken as a supplement, PS can be little short of miraculous as a way to boost your memory, improve your concentration, and brighten your mood. It's particularly helpful for improving short-term memory in older adults, as shown by a study of 149 people age fifty or older with "normal" age-related memory loss. Some of the study participants took 100 mg of PS three times a day for twelve weeks; the rest took a placebo. At the end of the experiment, the PS group showed a 15 percent improvement in learning and memory tasks. The greatest improvement was in the people who were the most impaired when they entered the study. Interestingly, the benefits continued for up to four weeks after the participants stopped taking PS.[7]

PS can also help prevent brain damage and other damage from excessive cortisol production. In a recent study of people who exercised intensely, PS kept cortisol levels from rising sharply.[8] Even if you don't exercise a lot, anything that keeps your brain from being bombarded by cortisol will help preserve your cognitive function.

Some recent research suggests that PS has a beneficial effect on all aspects of cell metabolism throughout your body. I'll be watching this research very carefully. If it continues to be promising, I think I'll be recommending PS as an all-around age-defying therapy.

Phosphatidyl serine is found naturally in many common foods, but only in very small amounts. And lecithin, containing the phospholipid phosphatidyl choline, which I'll discuss a few paragraphs down, doesn't have enough PS to raise your body levels in any significant way. To get the amounts you need to improve cognition, you need to take PS in supplement form.

Until recently, that was a somewhat chancy proposition, because PS supplements were made from cow brains and carried a very slight risk of viral infection. Today, however, PS supplements are made from soybeans and are quite safe. I recommend taking anywhere from 100 to 300 mg a day, preferably just before a meal. As the study of the fifty-and-overs suggested, the effects of supplemental PS continue for up to four weeks after you stop taking it. So if you are concerned about the cost of PS, which at the present writing is about a dollar for 100 mg, you can taper down the dosage once you have achieved a maximum apparent benefit. Cutting back to perhaps 60 to 100 mg daily at that point is fine for sustaining the brain-enhancing effect.

Because PS is a fat, it's vulnerable to free radical damage as it circulates in your body on its way to your brain. By following the entire age-defying protocol, which includes lots of antioxidant nutrients, you should have no trouble protecting the investment you're making in mental maintenance.

CHOLINE

Choline, a member of the B vitamin family, is needed to make the phospholipid phosphatidyl choline, or leci-

thin; it's also needed to make the neurotransmitter acetylcholine. At the Atkins Center, we use choline as part
of our treatment for estrogen-based disorders, heart disease, and some neurological problems such as Hunting-
ton's disease.

Choline has recently gained a reputation as a useful
overall memory-booster. A choline supplement called
DMAE (sometimes called deaner) is available, and it
may be the best version of choline to use. In animal
studies, DMAE has been shown to improve memory and
learning capacity, perhaps by raising phosphatidyl choline levels in the animals' brains. Even though there are
few studies showing that it works in humans, I have had
several patients who insist that DMAE has helped their
brain function. But please don't overlook the best dietary
source of phosphatidyl choline: egg yolks.

DOCOSAHEXAENOIC ACID (DHA)

Another major building block for brain cell membranes
is docosahexaenoic acid, better known as DHA. We
know that infants and young children need to get plenty
of DHA from their food for their rapidly growing brains
to develop fully. Today, there's increasing evidence to
show that DHA is essential for mental functioning in all
stages of life, from infancy to old age.

DHA is actually an omega-3 fatty acid that you get
from your food. Like EPA, another important omega-3
fatty acid, it's found primarily in cold-water fish such as
salmon and cod. If chickens are fed well, their egg yolks
can also be a great source of DHA. And, if you take
EPA supplements, you get a fair amount of DHA as
well. You could also try the newer DHA capsules that
are very low in EPA.

We have just begun to use higher doses of DHA at the Atkins Center, and we are already hearing some gratifying feedback from patients taking doses in the 500-mg range.

ACETYL-L-CARNITINE

The amino acid carnitine is one of my favorite vitanutrients. I use it extensively to treat heart disease and metabolic resistance to weight loss, and as a reliable nutritional answer to fatigue.

Acetyl-l-carnitine (ALC) is a sort of super-carnitine. In many ways, it's very similar to carnitine, but its molecular structure makes it easier to absorb, and it is much more focused on benefiting your brain. It can improve memory and alertness, slow the aging of brain cells, and energize your entire nervous system. A number of studies have shown that ALC can even slow the mental decline that comes with Alzheimer's disease and other forms of dementia.[9] Nor is it just for the elderly—ALC enhances mental performance in everyone, even twentysomethings.

It does this, generally speaking, by enhancing the ability of your cells to produce energy, and it manages that goal by transporting fat molecules into the mitochondria, where they can be burned as fuel. While it's there in the mitochondria, ALC also functions as a potent antioxidant that snuffs out free radicals as soon as they're created. In your brain, ALC is a crucial part of the process for creating the neurotransmitter acetylcholine. And, as discussed in Chapter 12, ALC also counteracts the aging effects of excess cortisol.

In your body, natural processes convert carnitine to the acetyl-l form, but only in small amounts. For the most effective ALC supplementation, therefore, carnitine supplements alone won't do the trick—ALC supplements will be much more effective. If you're a generally healthy person over forty, taking 500 to 1,000 mg of ALC daily will help improve your mental performance. As an added benefit, the ALC supplements will also raise your overall carnitine level. One word of caution: ALC invigorates your brain so well that it could keep you from sleeping. Take your ALC supplements in the morning.

PREGNENOLONE

Back in Chapter 12, I discussed the many uses of the grandmother hormone pregnenolone. Here I'll focus just on how pregnenolone can reverse age-related declines in memory and improve mental performance.

Pregnenolone works by enhancing your ability to transmit impulses from neuron to neuron. The faster and more efficiently the impulses travel, the better your brain works. Studies with lab animals show that even very small doses of pregnenolone markedly improve the animals' ability to learn and remember.[10] Very similar results have recently been documented in humans, where pregnenolone has been shown to improve memory in older adults as measured by standard memory tests.[11] In my experience, patients who take pregnenolone for reasons other than memory enhancement still report feeling sharper and more focused. Those who take it specifically *for* memory improvement notice definite improvements.

A daily pregnenolone dose of up to 100 mg should be sufficient to notice an uptick in your mental function.

THE B VITAMINS

The entire B vitamin complex—from thiamin through cobalamin, or vitamin B_{12}—is essential for proper brain function. Among other effects, all the B vitamins are required to make neurotransmitters, the chemical messengers that transmit impulses along your nerves and among your brain cells. If you're low on any one of the B vitamins, you're very likely to be low on the others as well. Even a very mild deficiency of any of the B vitamins is enough to cause such cognitive problems as memory loss, confusion, anxiety, depression, and sleep disorders.

I believe that deficiencies of B vitamins are an often overlooked cause of many cases of so-called senile dementia. The B vitamins in general are difficult to absorb from food. As we get older, our bodies have an even harder time taking them in. Combine that with the fact that many older people don't take in enough calories, and that the calories they do take in often come from foods low in B vitamins to begin with, and you practically have a formula for deficiency.

I've discussed the value of all the B vitamins at length in other writings.* Here I'll discuss just two of them in detail. The first is the one B vitamin that anyone over age fifty is most likely to be deficient in: cobalamin, also known as vitamin B_{12}. The second is folic acid, the B vitamin that protects not just your heart but also your brain.

Your level of vitamin B_{12} is seriously affected by aging. That's because to absorb B_{12} from your food, your

*Please see *Dr. Atkins' Vita-Nutrient Solution* for details.

stomach uses not only its usual hydrochloric acid and pepsin but also a special substance called intrinsic factor. As you age, however, you progressively make less and less of all your digestive fluids, including intrinsic factor. If you're over age sixty, there's a 50–50 chance that you're no longer making enough intrinsic factor to absorb all the vitamin B_{12} you need from your food. The result is the slow, insidious development of a B_{12} deficiency, along with symptoms of "senility." A serious B_{12} deficiency shows up easily on a blood test, because it causes a very obvious type of anemia. Mild B_{12} deficiency isn't visible on a blood test, however, and older people who are just on the low end of normal can still show symptoms of deficiency.

In fact, the prevalance of vitamin B_{12} deficiency among older adults is startlingly high. According to a recent study, some 40 percent of the population over age sixty-seven has suboptimal levels, and 12 percent have outright deficiency.[12]

Many mainstream physicians are aware that their elderly patients may well be low in vitamin B_{12} and routinely administer B_{12} shots to them. There's a better way. A B_{12} deficiency develops slowly, often starting years before your doctor would consider you elderly. The damage it causes happens gradually and can't always be reversed. Much better to start taking B_{12} now. I recommend to all my patients, no matter their age, that they keep their brains sharp by taking B_{12} supplements. For patients under age forty, I recommend 1,000 mcg a day. Between age forty and sixty, 200 mcg daily is good insurance. After age sixty, the age-defying dosage should go up to 400 mcg. Your vitamin B_{12} level should still be checked regularly; the dosage may well need to be increased as you get older.

Earlier in this book, I discussed how important folic

acid is to the health of your heart (see Chapter 4). The benefits also apply to your brain, and for the same reason. Folic acid lowers the amount of artery-damaging homocysteine in your blood. That helps prevent not just heart attacks but also strokes and reduced cerebral circulation from hardened arteries in the brain. The evidence? Alzheimer's patients, to take just one example, tend to have low blood levels of both folic acid and vitamin B_{12}, along with moderately elevated blood levels of homocysteine. In a recent study, researchers looked at homocysteine levels in two groups of people over age fifty-five—one group that had Alzheimer's disease and one that didn't. The people with the highest level of homocysteine were 4.5 times more likely to have Alzheimer's than those with the lowest level. Similarly, those with the lowest level of folic acid were 3.3 times more likely to have Alzheimer's, while those with the lowest vitamin B_{12} level were 4.3 times more likely to have it.[13]

The B vitamins may also help you hear, and hearing loss is a very common and underdiagnosed problem among adults over fifty. The biological mechanisms that cause age-related hearing impairment are unknown, but there's a good chance that deficiencies of folic acid and vitamin B_{12} play a major part. In one recent study of healthy older women, the ones with impaired hearing had 38 percent lower blood levels of vitamin B_{12} and 31 percent lower levels of folic acid than women with normal hearing.[14]

As I complained back in Chapter 4, even though the FDA has mandated that processed-grain foods like bread, baked goods, and breakfast cereal now contain supplemental folic acid, the official recommended daily intake is still only a pitiful 800 mcg. I believe that is far too low to have an adequate positive effect on your health. I suggest that basically healthy people take in at least 3 to 8 mg (3,000–8,000 mcg) a day—more with a family history of age-related hearing loss, heart disease, stroke, or early senility.

"SMART DRUGS" AND THE SAMe PROMISES

With longevity looking more possible for more people than ever before, antiaging panaceas are being developed thick and fast. Because I have a reputation as an "alternative" doctor, hardly a day goes by without my getting promotional material about some new "smart drug" or fabulous new supplement that's supposed to enhance your brain power and reverse the aging process.

One of the hottest new antiaging supplements today is S-adenosylmethionine, better known as SAMe. At the Atkins Center, we have used this natural version of the amino acid methionine mainly as a safe, drug-free treatment for depression, but now there may be another reason to prescribe SAMe.

Recent research shows that Alzheimer's patients have very low SAMe levels in their brains. This was something of a surprise to the researchers, because earlier studies had shown that these patients had high levels of SAMe—but in their blood. There still haven't been any studies of whether supplemental SAMe will help slow Alzheimer's disease.[15]

Is SAMe helpful for ordinary brain aging? It's simply too early to tell.

In addition to SAMe, I'm familiar with much of the research into the so-called "smart drugs"; the research is being carried out primarily in Europe, where I have wide-ranging contacts with colleagues. Some of these drugs do indeed have merit, but I don't prescribe them often, mainly because the vitanutrients I've talked about in this chapter seem to benefit so many of my patients so well. The drugs' benefits are generally outweighed by their drawbacks, expense, and unavailability: Most of these medications aren't readily available in the United States, even though they're sometimes sold over-the-counter in Europe.

But be aware that such smart drugs as deprenyl, hydergine, vinpocetin, piracetam, and others are not do-it-yourself medicine. They are prescription drugs, not dietary supplements, and there are risks to using them. You need to work closely with a physician who is accustomed to using these drugs. Even then, I feel strongly that the same benefits can be achieved through nutrition, with less trouble and expense, with far less risk—and more effectively.

With this chapter, we put a finish to what we might describe as the top part of the recipe for defying age— the list of ingredients. You now know what you need to counter the effects of aging and how each ingredient works. It's time to put it all together into a program that will help you stay healthy and active over a very long lifetime.

19

CREATING YOUR AGE-DEFYING DIET

What does it take to defy age and counter the effects of the so-called "aging process"? It takes a program combining the right diet, the right set of vitanutrients, and the right kinds of exercise done regularly. It must be a program you can and will make part of your life, so it must be easy to follow and comfortable to do. In the next five chapters, you're going to learn how to create your own age-defying program.

We'll start here by discussing the concepts for creating the age-defying diet. In the chapters that follow, we'll discuss the kinds of foods that form the age-defying diet and the principles or guidelines by which you can put those foods together into a personal diet plan. In Chapter 22, we'll add the specific vitanutrient supplements that are right for you and for the health issues that concern you. Finally, we'll see how to put all of these program elements together so you stay healthy and prevent the degenerative diseases of aging.

But before we do any of that, let's review the foundation of the age-defying diet. Some of you, in fact, may just be starting to read this book at this point. For you as well, here's a reexamination of what we've learned in the earlier parts of this book and what we can conclude from what we've learned.

First of all, we discussed some basic facts about why we age. Here's some of what we learned:

- The greatest inhibitor of a full life span is atherosclerosis—having your vital arteries blocked by plaque.
- Atherosclerosis is a condition of our distorted modern diet, one that has been in existence (except in rare, isolated cases) for only about seventy-five years.
- Atherosclerosis is part and parcel of an insulin disorder—excessive insulin—that develops mainly among people who consume a diet made up mostly of refined carbohydrates, especially junk carbohydrates such as white flour, sugar, and corn syrup.
- The insulin disorder leads to unhealthy elevations of blood glucose, a characteristic of diabetes and related disorders. Elevations of glucose in turn lead inexorably to premature aging by creating AGEs—advanced glycosylation end-products—created when the extra sugar in your system combines with essential body proteins.
- Insulin, the hormone that naturally brings our sugar levels down, is extremely atherogenic—that is, a major cause of atherosclerosis.
- Logically, the best way to avoid the glucose-versus-insulin dilemma is to follow a low-glycemic diet—a diet that is the least able to raise your glucose and insulin levels.
- Because carbohydrates are all, to some extent, glycemic, and because noncarbohydrate foods are barely glycemic at all, a low-carbohydrate diet—the best way to achieve a low-glycemic diet—will correct the most prevalent cause of

atherosclerosis, as my patients have proved over
and over again.

- If you're overweight, a low-carbohydrate diet
causes an automatic loss of weight by switching
your primary source of energy fuel to stored
body fat. If your weight is normal or below normal, however, the low-carbohydrate diet must be
modified so that you prevent the production of
excess insulin while maintaining your weight.

Put all the above together and you have a pretty clear
idea of the first essential point of any age-defying diet:
*No matter what your weight, you must reduce the
amount of refined carbohydrates in your diet.* And if you
do need to lose weight, the low-carbohydrate diet is the
best, easiest, safest, and most luxurious way to do it.

Let me be perfectly clear about this: The age-defying
diet, like my weight-loss diet, is a low-carbohydrate diet.
It is *not* a low-calorie diet. You will never have to go
hungry, much less starve yourself, on any diet I suggest.

But there is more we can do to defy age than just
limit carbohydrates. Other facts examined in earlier
chapters led us to a second important conclusion about
what constitutes an age-defying diet.

- Most theorists on aging agree that free radical
activity is a primary cause of the symptoms of
aging. Nutritional antioxidants play a well-
established, proven role in preventing aging.
- Antioxidants from food may prove more valuable than the antioxidants given as nutritional
supplements. Vegetables and fruits contain significant amounts of antioxidant flavonoids and
other beneficial phytochemicals—so many that

we haven't begun to identify them all yet. Supplements are often needed to give you an extra antioxidant boost, but drinking green tea and eating plenty of fresh vegetables and low-sugar fruits gives you the best variety of flavonoids.

• There is a wide disparity in nutritional value and glucose content even among foods in the same category. Among the fruits, for instance, bananas are little more than unwanted carbohydrates, but blueberries are relatively low in sugar and very high in antioxidants. The *quality* of your food selections assumes paramount importance.

Put all this together, and you've got the second essential point of your antiaging diet: *You need a diet that is high in antioxidants, primarily from fresh vegetables and low-sugar fruits—and from supplements as needed.*

An antiaging diet, therefore, must be low in carbohydrates and high in antioxidants. But there's one more very important factor in creating such a diet: We are all individuals, with different genetic predispositions, different histories, different health problems to overcome, different tastes in food, and different metabolic responses. *Therefore, one diet cannot fit all.*

What's more, while diet alone will make a big difference in how you age, we also need to remember three other components that fend off the symptoms of aging: hormones, brain nutrients, and exercise.

Bottom line: When we put all these factors and conclusions together, we can create a diet that *will* help slow the aging process and keep you in the best possible mental and physical health.

PLANNING YOUR AGE-DEFYING DIET

What is *your* age-defying diet? That's what we're going
to create. I cannot give you a one-size-fits-all Atkins
Age-Defying Diet that works for everybody and promises you'll live for a century. But I can and will do for
you what I do for each patient who sees me privately in
consultation: *I will teach you basic dietary principles
and help you select an eating program that best meets
your needs and your health profile.*

Your personal program will be based on the age-
defying diet principles I've learned from years of studying the research and attending and speaking at hundreds
of medical conferences around the world. Most of all,
my age-defying principles are based on the experience
I've gained from treating more than 60,000 patients over
forty years.

UNDOING THE DAMAGE

My first age-defying principle is very straightforward.
You must undo the damage you've suffered from the
dietary mistakes Western culture has perpetrated in the
twentieth century.

As a first step, you'll need to unlearn the biggest mis-
take of all—the so-called "food pyramid." In the more
than ten years since this dietary fraud was foisted on the
public by our own government, Americans have become
fatter than ever. Why? Because the food pyramid is
heavily based on carbohydrates of the worst sort: refined
grains in the form of bread, pasta, rice, and similar foods.
(Not coincidentally, in my opinion, these foods are also

the ones that are most profitable for the big food processors.) The food pyramid tells you that protein is bad and fat is worse.

Ignore the food pyramid and the entrenched medical/financial interests that push it. Improve your health and prolong your life by cutting carbohydrates from your diet to the degree that is appropriate for you.

CARBOHYDRATE COMPREHENSION

To find the right level of carbohydrates for you, you'll need to understand your own metabolism. If you are overweight, you need to get below your critical carbohydrate level for losing—your CCLL. You need to stay at that level until you are at your ideal weight. Then you need to find your critical carbohydrate level for maintenance—your CCLM. Once you've discovered your maintenance carbohydrate level, you need to stay at it for life. I'm not condemning you to a lifetime of dieting and being hungry—I'm helping you make a lifestyle change that will give you better health, more energy, and a longer life.

If your weight is normal, concern yourself with the nature of your carbohydrates. Most of the carbohydrates you eat should be both complex and unrefined. What does that mean?

Complex carbohydrates are basically starchy foods—including whole grains; vegetable carbohydrates like butternut squash, potatoes, and sweet potatoes; and legumes such as lentils, peas, and beans. (As a bonus, legumes are also a good source of vegetable protein.)

Vegetables qualify as unrefined, but not all grains do. The term "unrefined" refers to whole grains that haven't been so overprocessed that they have no nutritional value. Foods made with unrefined whole grains are hard to come by. The brown-colored commercial bread that passes for "healthy" whole wheat is definitely not what I mean. If you look at the ingredients label, you'll see that these foods are still made mostly from refined white flour. I'll tell you more about the value of whole grains and the best ways to get them in your diet in a subsequent chapter.

Simple carbohydrates are sugars—glucose, sucrose, fructose, lactose, maltose, and so on. Sugars are found in a lot of common foods: milk (lactose), fruit (fructose), beer (maltose), table sugar, sweets, baked goods like cake and cookies (sucrose), and soft drinks (corn syrup). These foods have a very high glycemic index—meaning that the sugars enter your bloodstream quite quickly—and that can send your insulin level soaring. It is essential that you keep simple carbohydrates to the barest possible minimum in your diet. Simple carbohydrates should make up no more than 15 percent of your daily carbohydrate intake. If your daily carbs are no more than 20 percent of your daily diet, that means that simple carbohydrates should be no more than 15 percent of 20 percent, or about 3 percent of your daily total. If you must eat something sweet, make it a low-sugar fresh fruit whenever possible. (I'll explain more about how to avoid simple carbohydrates and give you a list of the best fruits to eat in Chapter 21.)

Keep refined carbs—flours, sugars, corn syrup—to a minimum, less than one serving daily. That means cutting back sharply on foods like pasta, bread, rice, and baked goods, to say nothing of candy and soda pop. I'd be the first to admit that's a big change in diet for most people. But I can also tell you that the very foods that you think you can't live without are the ones that will shorten your life. The millions of people who follow my diet plan have gladly given up these foods in exchange for losing weight and finding improved health. Do you love jelly donuts so much that you're willing to trade ten years of your life for them? Ask yourself that—ask your family that—and then change the way you eat.

CARBOHYDRATES FOR UNSTABLE BLOOD SUGAR

When you digest your food, both simple and complex carbohydrates are converted into glucose, your body's primary energy fuel. But the conversion process happens at different speeds. Complex carbs, especially if they're also high in dietary fiber, take a while to be digested and converted. When you eat these foods, the glucose is released into your blood slowly and steadily. As your blood sugar slowly rises, your pancreas slowly releases insulin to carry the glucose into your cells. That's why we say these foods have a low glycemic index—the glucose enters your bloodstream slowly.

Sugars, however, are much simpler to digest. They have a very high glycemic index, meaning they enter your bloodstream almost as soon as you swallow them. To cope with the sudden onslaught, your pancreas has to release a lot of insulin all at once. All that insulin mops up all the extra blood glucose so efficiently that your glucose level falls sharply.

If your body can handle glucose normally, and if you eat a mixed meal that includes a variety of foods, the effects on your blood sugar of eating some simple carbohydrates will be relatively benign. Your body will cope efficiently with the unneeded sugar, and your blood sugar and insulin levels will return to their normal levels smoothly—for now. As you get older and continue to eat this way, however, your body may become less and less efficient at dealing with the extra glucose.

Unfortunately, nearly half the adults over the age of forty in the United States can't handle glucose normally. I base this estimate on the incidence of Type II (adult-onset) diabetes, which is about 8 percent of the total population and 16 percent of those over forty. Those are the people in whom diabetes has been detected; easily as many people have undiagnosed diabetes. People with abnormal glucose metabolism outnumber full-fledged diabetics by about three to one.

If you're one of those people with abnormal glucose metabolism—and chances are good you are, especially if you're overweight—your blood glucose levels have roller-coaster ups and downs. You get all the symptoms of unstable blood sugar, including variable energy levels, mood swings, and such cognition problems as fuzzy thinking or brain fog. If the symptoms come on when you are hungry and are relieved by eating, then unstable blood sugar is almost certainly the culprit.

Do not, by the way, let your conventional doctor do a simple blood test for high blood sugar and tell you that you're fine. The only way to learn if you have unstable blood sugar is to have a full, five-hour glucose tolerance test administered by a doctor who knows what he or she is doing.

Your blood sugar is destabilized by carbohydrates. It's basically unaffected by protein, and it's stabilized by dietary fats and oils. If unstable blood sugar is a problem for you, a diet low in carbohydrates and reasonably high in fat may help normalize it. This fact, plus the fact that scientific researchers keep demonstrating that dietary fats actually contribute to good health, allows me to recommend to my patients with symptoms of unstable blood sugar a diet in which 50 percent of the total calories are consumed as fat. When they eat a high-fat diet, they invariably get better.

FAT FACTS

An essential component of your antiaging diet is avoidance of the unhealthy fats that have been brought into widespread use in the last century. As discussed in detail back in Chapter 14, I'm not talking about the saturated fats, such as butter and animal fat, that your conventional doctor considers unhealthy. I mean the deadly trans fats that are now found in all sorts of foods, including the margarine your conventional doctor recommends instead of butter.

Trans fats, not saturated fats, are the dietary link to elevated cholesterol and heart disease. Trans fats lower HDL cholesterol, raise LDL cholesterol, increase lipoprotein(a), and elevate total cholesterol by 20 to 30 percent. In addition, trans fats reduce your responsiveness to insulin and block your uptake of the essential fatty acids you need for good health.

SELECT SAFE FOODS

Most of the prepared and processed foods we eat today are designed for long shelf life rather than for good nutrition. The nutrients originally present in the fresh version of these foods have virtually been eliminated—replaced with preservatives, food colorings, and all sorts of additives. Avoid these foods. Select unprocessed foods whenever possible. And watch out for "low-fat" foods—the fats in these foods have been replaced by carbohydrates.

Make sure that the majority of animal foods you eat do not contain hormones or antibiotics. Choose hormone-free, antibiotic-free, organic meats and free-range poultry and eggs whenever possible. I realize that these options are not always available, especially in restaurants. But try to avoid foods from animals that have been fed hormones or antibiotics.

Today, of course, hormone-treated beef is a major international trade issue. European countries have quite rightly banned the import of this meat from America. Rather than rethinking the issue examining the evidence of how unhealthy beef treated in this way is, American trade officials have been fighting the ban in every way they can. It's the food establishment at work again, this time with the overt support of your government, to keep you from getting safe food unless you're willing to pay a premium price for organic meat.

Avoid, too, genetically modified and irradiated foods. Foods that have been irradiated have longer shelf lives but sharply reduced nutrition. Irradiation destroys valuable phytochemicals in plant foods, and it destroys vitamins in all foods. Meats that have been irradiated are not only less nutritious, they're also far less flavorful. In my opinion, it's a crime to take a delicious rib-eye steak and turn it into a mushy, tasteless lump by irradiating it.

Genetically modified foods are the latest trend in agribusiness. Genetic modification goes far beyond traditional plant breeding to improve the characteristics of the crop. By inserting genes from other species altogether into the basic genome of a plant, genetic engineers are creating "improved" varieties that have a lot of potential dangers. Among other problems, these foods are a real risk to people with food allergies. A genetically modified plant that contains a peanut gene, for instance, could trigger a serious reaction in someone allergic to peanuts. Fortunately, consumer acceptance of genetically modified food in the United States is still low. In Europe, there is a strong movement to ban these products.

GETTING THE MOST FROM YOUR MEALS

So many of our foods today have been so heavily processed that they contain calories but not nutrition. Even many fresh fruits and vegetables have been bred for ease of handling and storage and no longer have high nutrient levels or good taste. By the time they arrive at your supermarket from factory farms in other parts of the country, they have lost what nutritive value they had. Just think of the typical supermarket tomato, and you'll know what I mean.

You need to make the most of your meals by choosing nutrient-dense foods. That means foods that have been minimally processed; are high in vitamins, minerals, and phytochemicals; and have little or no pesticide, hormone, or antibiotic content.

Choose the freshest foods you can find, preferably from local suppliers and organic growers. The difference in nutrient density when you buy fresh local produce is sometimes remarkable. Whenever I go to Greece, for example, I'm always amazed at the eggs. When they're cooked sunny-side up, the yolks are a magnificent deep yellow-orange color. They're almost too beautiful to eat. I eat them with relish, though, because they taste delicious and because they have ten times the amount of the vital brain nutrient DHA as do eggs produced on an American factory farm. But even here in the United States, if you buy organic, free-range eggs from a local farmer, you'll be getting much more nutrition and better taste.

VARIETY IS THE SPICE OF HEALTH

Despite all my criticisms of the American food industry, it is true that it has made a wide variety of fresh foods available all year round. Today we can easily achieve tremendous variety in our diets. There are two reasons why this can help us.

First, each food is capable of providing us with a different lineup of vitanutrients, thus enhancing the breadth of all food-based nutrition. We know that the phytochemicals in plant foods are very valuable, but we haven't identified them all yet. By eating a variety of foods, you get the benefits of the full range of phytochemicals. Second, eating the same food repeatedly has been shown to create a high incidence of intolerance, or even addiction, to that very food.

Many of my medical colleagues report that they can help the majority of their patients simply by prescribing a "rotational diet." On this diet, patients eat a particular food—cottage cheese, say—only once every three days. Then they wait. It's a little like the pitching rotation in major league baseball, so patients know when it's the turn of cottage cheese again.

FEND OFF FOOD ALLERGIES

Hidden food intolerances or food allergies are one of the most common health problems we deal with at the Atkins Center. It's important that you discover any food intolerances or allergies you may have and eliminate those foods from your diet.

These food intolerances often develop simply from

eating the same food too often. Sometimes, the food intolerance becomes fixed enough that it takes several months of eliminating the food from the diet before the intolerance is "cured." In the case of true allergies, the restriction might be permanent.

You can begin to discover your own food intolerances simply by being alert to your reactions to various foods. An often repeated example is the drowsiness many of my patients feel after eating a grain food containing wheat or gluten.

To learn more about any food intolerances or allergies you have, you'll need to work with a physician, generally one who practices complementary medicine. The best way to diagnose intolerances is with a blood specimen using the cytotoxic test or the ALCAT. You'll need to modify your diet based on the results.

ASSESSING YOUR PAST DIET

The final step to take in planning how to create your own age-defying diet is to analyze your previous dietary history from the vantage point of the information in this book. If you have spent your life eating a lot of junk food or avoiding foods you now know to be contributors to good health, the moment has come to start making up the difference. Try to compensate by developing the habit of eating differently enough to correct your previous diet's excesses or inadequacies. That's what I'll be talking about in the next few chapters.

20

THE AGE-DEFYING DIET: THE BASICS

At the Atkins Center, we have long worked with two basic sets of dietary instructions. The instructions are flexible enough that we can individualize them for each patient, but basically, one diet induces weight loss—regardless of the amount of food consumed—while the other does not.

This latter diet, the one that is suitable for people who do not have overt blood sugar or weight problems, will serve as the fulcrum and, in a sense, the benchmark of the basic age-defying diet principles that are the subject of this chapter. Now that you understand the basic components of a nutrition plan, these principles will guide you to form your own plan.

The diet that does *not* induce weight loss at present applies to only a minority of Americans, since more than half of us are overweight. If the message of this book is heeded, however, in the future the non-weight-loss diet will apply to most of us, especially those who are fortunate enough to be started early on the principles this chapter discusses. Why are such people particularly fortunate? Because from an early age, they will be eating in a way that prevents blood sugar problems, high blood pressure, and obesity. Interestingly, they will be eating the foods Americans ate more than a century ago, before heart attacks were ever heard of.

But perhaps you're wondering why you should go on a diet if you don't need to lose weight. Because like practically all Americans, even those of normal weight, you are at grave risk of developing blood sugar problems later on, if you're not on the brink of such problems already. The reason is the typical junk-focused American diet, which is far too high in refined carbohydrates and far too low in healthy fats, oils, and protein.

For example, if you've been faithfully following the government-approved food pyramid for "healthy" eating, you are more than likely to develop unstable blood sugar. The pyramid's diet calls for you to eat six to eleven servings a day of refined grains like bread, pasta, and cereals—the junk-food equivalent of swallowing two cups of pure table sugar. That's on top of the 150 pounds of sugar or corn syrup per year—nearly one cup a day—that are typically part of the average American's diet.

As you know from reading the earlier chapters of this book, nothing will age your body and mind faster than excess glucose in your blood. By following the healthy, natural, insulin-regulating diet that I'm teaching you, you will, over the long run, keep your blood sugar and insulin levels under control and forestall or even prevent premature aging and serious health problems. And that's why you're reading this book.

YOUR GOAL: STABLE BLOOD SUGAR

My age-defying diet is based on integrating twin objectives. One is to employ a diet that corrects the metabolic vulnerabilities that apply uniquely to each individual. The other objective is to endow the diet amply with the vitanutrients most useful in fighting off aging changes.

The first objective is best met by stabilizing your blood sugar. Put it this way: You enjoy optimal health only when your sugar level stays in an optimal range. You can achieve stable blood sugar by replacing most simple carbohydrates and sugar-containing foods with either complex carbohydrates or noncarbohydrate food. One result is that you will likely be eating more protein and fats than you're accustomed to. But they are there to stabilize your blood sugar and provide the nutritionally essential amino acids and fatty acids that are as indispensable to you as vitamins and minerals.

The second objective of my age-defying diet is best met by a diet that is low in foods that create free radicals and high in the antioxidants that fight them. To reduce your intake of radical-producing foods, the diet eliminates sugar and trans fats—like margarine—from your diet. To increase your antioxidant capacity, the diet emphasizes fresh vegetables and such low-sugar fruits as berries.

The great beauty of the age-defying diet is that it is very easy to stick to. It's delicious, you never have to count calories, and you don't need to keep track of portion size. You'll enjoy all the steaks and lobster you want, along with unlimited quantities of fresh vegetables and satisfying whole grains.

True, unhealthy sugary foods like cake and cookies are now permanently out the window, but in their place is a variety of fresh fruits, as well as desserts made with natural noncaloric substances that are actually much sweeter than sugar. My patients invariably tell me that they lose their taste for sugary foods once they've been on the diet for a couple of weeks. They soon find that typical snacks and desserts taste almost disgustingly sweet.

On the antiaging diet, your consumption of refined complex carbohydrates like white rice, bread, and pasta is also very limited. In their place, however, are highly nutritious, highly flavorful whole grains like brown rice and genuine whole-grain bread. As with sugary foods, once you start eating whole grains you will soon lose your taste for pasty, flavorless foods made with refined grains.

THE COMPONENTS OF THE AGE-DEFYING DIET

The age-defying diet has three components: proteins and fat, complex carbohydrates, and simple carbohydrates. Let's sort the most common foods into their categories and the proportions these foods should contribute to your overall diet:

Protein and fats: Meat, poultry, eggs, fish, seafood, cheese, nuts, seeds, olives, avocados, fats and oils. The range is 50 to 75 percent.

Complex carbohydrates: Vegetables, grains, whole-grain flour products (pasta, for instance), and legumes (beans). The range is 25 to 50 percent (the lower end is more desirable).

Simple carbohydrates: Fruit, fruit juice, sweets (sugar, honey, maple syrup, etc.), milk, yogurt. The range is less than 10 percent. Whole fruits that are low in sugar content (berries, melons, peaches, plums, apricots, kiwis, and so on) should make up the majority of this category.

Now let's take them one component at a time.

Proteins and Fats

To achieve the desirable protein and fat percentages on the age-defying diet, animal foods—meat, poultry, fish, and shellfish—are all permitted in unlimited quantities. Canned fish such as sardines, salmon, and tuna are fine, but be careful of processed meats like frankfurters and cold cuts. Many of these foods contain hidden carbohydrates in the form of milk solids or corn syrup as fillers and flavoring. They're also full of undesirable chemical additives like MSG and nitrates. Just as bad are meats filled with added hormones and antibiotics. To avoid these dangerous additives, whenever possible select "organic" meats. Many meats imported from Argentina or New Zealand are thus qualified.

Eggs are also permitted without restriction. Eat the whole egg, not just the whites. As I've pointed out over and over again in this book, eggs are the perfect protein food and contain numerous nutrients that are valuable to your health.

Cheeses are permitted without restriction (except for people on a diet to control yeast overgrowth), because the processing sharply reduces the amount of lactose, or milk sugar, in these dairy products. Be sure you're eating real cheese, and not a processed cheese food like Velveeta or American cheese that contains corn oil instead of butterfat.

Milk and yogurt are high in lactose, a simple sugar, and should be kept to a minimum on the antiaging diet. In addition, a significant part of the population can't digest lactose properly or is allergic to milk—another good reason to cut down on these foods. Consume no more than one cup of milk daily. Lactose-reduced milk, by the way, has almost exactly the same carbohydrate content as whole milk. If you enjoy yogurt and can digest it easily, eat no more than one cup daily, and eat only the plain, live-culture variety. An eight-ounce container of low-fat, fruit-flavored yogurt contains seven teaspoons of added sugar.

Cream is allowed—in fact, I encourage you to use it. Cream contains very little lactose and is an excellent source of dietary fat. Never use nondairy creamers or lighteners. These artificial substances are nothing but sweetened chemicals.

All nuts and seeds are permitted. I particularly recommend macadamia nuts. These tasty, crunchy nuts are high in fat and low in carbohydrates. They're the perfect snack food. Other good nut choices are pecans, filberts, and walnuts. Nut butters are permitted, but only if they contain no added sweeteners or partially hydrogenated vegetable oils. That leaves out many commercial peanut butters. Check your local health food store for nut butters with no additives.

Fats and oils are nutritionally essential, no matter what the American Heart Association and the rest of the medical establishment tell you. They should never be avoided or feared—with one exception. That's the dangerous trans fats I talked about back in Chapter 14. If the label on the food container says "partially hydrogenated vegetable oil," stay away. Your conventional doctor may well have told you to stop eating butter and to switch to healthier margarine. Don't you believe it! Exactly the opposite is true.

In fact, let's go through it once more: Margarine is nothing but trans fats. Eating this stuff promises to release cascades of artery-damaging free radicals in your body. Butter doesn't do this. It not only gives your food a richer, more satisfying taste, it is also a rather safe form of fat. All fats, butter included, help stabilize your blood sugar.

For salads and cooking, such monounsaturated vegetable oils as olive, almond, avocado, and macadamia are ideal. Cold-pressed polyunsaturated vegetable oils like walnut, soy, sesame, sunflower, and safflower are also fine. These oils are excellent dietary sources of omega-3 and omega-6 essential fatty acids. Skip the corn oil and the canola oil—they're far too high in omega-6.

Complex Carbohydrates

We come now to that part of the age-defying diet that distinguishes it from the Atkins weight-loss diet. On the age-defying diet, we *allow* carbohydrates, but only those that contribute most to your health.

Start by replacing the simple carbohydrates in your diet—that is, the sugars—with high-quality complex carbohydrates—the starches. Simple sugars send your blood sugar crashing up and down. Complex carbohydrates are more likely to keep your blood sugar steady, especially when you combine them with protein and fat.

Notice my emphasis on the phrase "high-quality" when discussing complex carbohydrates. Foods such as white rice, pasta, and bread are, technically speaking, complex carbohydrates, but their *quality* is very low. The grains used to make these foods have been processed to the point of nutritional nonexistence. The phytochemicals and fiber in them have been removed, leaving behind nothing but refined, concentrated carbohydrates, which your body converts almost instantly to glucose. Yet in many cases, these foods have been mistakenly pushed upon us as health foods. As a result, they are overconsumed; one consequence is that they are frequently the objects of food intolerances.

The age-defying diet emphasizes the high-quality complex carbohydrates found in whole grains and vegetables. These foods are delicious, filling, and full of fiber, vitamins, minerals, and phytochemicals that fight free radicals and offer additional beneficial effects.

On the age-defying diet, if it's green, it's a relatively free food (unless you're better off on a really low-carbohydrate diet). This means go ahead and consume generous and varied portions of salad greens, broccoli, kale, Brussels sprouts, collard greens, green beans, and so on—as much as four to six cups a day.

Other vegetables—carrots, beets, peas, and squash, for example—are higher in carbohydrates, but they're also high in antioxidant carotenes and other nutrients (check back to Chapter 10 for more on carotenes). To get the benefits of the phytochemicals without overdoing the carbohydrates, refer to the tables in Chapter 21 and select those vegetables that provide significant amounts of phytochemcials without a major intake of carbohydrates.

Starchy vegetables, beans and legumes, corn, and even potatoes can be useful sources of vegetable protein, essential fatty acids, fiber, vitanutrients, and phytochemicals. On the other hand, because they are relatively high in starch that your body will convert to glucose, they could raise your blood sugar, especially if you tend even slightly in that direction. Because these foods are also high in fiber, however, the rise in blood sugar they cause is slower and far less dramatic than it would be if you ate an equivalent amount of a refined carbohydrate like pasta.

I find that my patients need to experiment a bit to find the level of complex carbohydrates that is right for them. In general, if you are of normal weight, limit starchy vegetables, potatoes, beans, and similar foods to one or two servings a day. However, if you find yourself losing weight on the age-defying diet, add another serving or two. People who are underweight should fill up on vegetables. This may include three to four servings of complex carbohydrates a day.

As you permanently change your eating habits, you'll discover the amount of complex carbohydrates that satisfies you and also keeps your weight and blood sugar at the appropriate level. You can even allow yourself the occasional little binge, as long as you stick to bingeing on high-quality carbohydrates. If you want to have a small serving of pasta, for instance, do so—as long as you make it whole-wheat pasta or buckwheat noodles. If you'd like some rice, brown rice is certainly better than white. And a small baked potato with the skin is far better than a serving of french fries.

Simple Carbohydrates

If you're overweight, I have a very simple method for determining how much simple carbohydrate to include in your diet. Just follow these easy steps: Take a piece of paper. Take a pencil. Draw a large circle on the paper. Read the answer. That's a zero.

If you're of normal weight, you still want to keep simple carbohydrates to a bare minimum, not to mention such highly refined complex carbohydrates as pasta, bread, and sugary foods. Not only are the simple-carb foods very high on the glycemic index, they're also heavily processed foods with very little nutritional value—the emptiest of empty calories.

What about fresh fruit? There is a place for it, but it is not the unrestricted benefactor many dietitians today believe it to be. Bear in mind that most of the calories in fruit come from the simple sugars, fructose and glucose, the very sugars present in white table sugar.

The other side of the coin, however, is that fruit is a useful source of fiber, vitamins, minerals, and phytochemicals. If you're of normal weight, fresh whole fruits in modest amounts can be acceptable, although you should learn which fruits provide the greatest phytochemical and vitanutrient intake in relation to their sugar content. Table 21.2 in Chapter 21 should help you make good selections. You will see that the greatest advantage comes from berries of all sorts, backed up by melons, peaches, plums, apricots, and kiwi.

Fruit juices are most assuredly not a good alternative to fruit and should be avoided. The juicing process removes the fiber and concentrates the sugar. As an example, take orange juice. For all the heavy advertising claiming it to be an excellent source of vitamin C, folic acid, potassium, and other vitanutrients, OJ is also extremely high in sugar. One eight-ounce serving contains more than 25 grams of sugar—more than the average candy bar. Apple juice, grape juice, pineapple juice, and prune juice all have even more.

Among the vegetable juices, carrot juice is very high in sugar and should be avoided. It would be appropriate only as a minor addition to mixed vegetable juices. On the other hand, tomato juice is definitely worth your effort. A six-ounce glass of tomato juice, even the processed kind out of the bottle, contains enough lycopene to make a difference.

Canned fruits have virtually no nutritional value, and they are loaded with added sugar. The same is true of dried fruit, such as dried pineapple. Sugar or some other sweetener is often added in the processing, even if the product is advertised as "healthy," "organic," or "natural."

As for other simple sugars, the short answer is no. The long answer is—if you're addicted to sweets—no. If you're not addicted to sweets, then you can have simple sugars once in a leap year blue moon. You need to avoid all caloric sweeteners, including table sugar, honey, maple syrup, corn syrup, fructose, maltose (found in beer, even the nonalcoholic kind), and lactose (milk sugar). Basically, if the food ends in *-ose*, it's a sugar and should be avoided.

If you feel the need for something sweet, select or create a rich dessert sweetened by a noncaloric sweetener. The two most desirable alternative sweeteners available today are stevia and sucralose.

Stevia is a natural plant product from South America that has been used safely worldwide for years. The stevia herb in its natural form is about ten to fifteen times sweeter than table sugar. Stevia extracts are much sweeter, some one hundred to three hundred times sweeter than table sugar, so a tiny bit goes a long way.

Sucralose has just been approved by the FDA for use in the United States. It is derived from table sugar, but sucralose is six hundred times sweeter. What's more, sucralose is absorbed into your body only in limited amounts. That means that your overworked insulin mechanism need not be involved.

A couple of years ago, the FDA, in one of its many misguided attempts to "protect" American consumers— and the corporate giant that manufactures aspartame— tried to force the publisher of a cookbook of stevia recipes to destroy them. Public outrage put a stop to the strong-arm tactics, but to this day stevia can be sold only in health food stores as a dietary supplement.

Stevia or sucralose is a much better choice for a noncaloric sweetener than aspartame, an artificial sweetener found in such products as Nutra-Sweet and Equal that often seems to cause side effects in many of my patients. In particular, my patients who drank three or more servings a day of aspartame-sweetened beverages seemed to have trouble losing weight and controlling their unstable blood sugar.

DRINK UP

Drinking sufficient fluids is an important aspect of the age-defying diet. Consume liquids liberally, but don't force yourself. Your goal should be to drink at least eight 8-ounce glasses of fluid a day. Plain, pure water is the most natural and best of all liquids to drink.

If possible, the water you drink should be bottled spring water, bottled mineral water, or tap water from an effective water filtration system. Plain sodium-free seltzer and essence-flavored unsweetened seltzers are also fine. You can make your own lemonade with fresh lemon juice, pure water, and a noncaloric sweetener like stevia.

Herbal teas, when made with pure water, are an enjoyable alternative to plain water. Choose herbal teas that are free of caffeine, added sweeteners, fruit, and barley malt. Good choices are peppermint, chamomile, and raspberry leaf.

Decaffeinated coffee and tea are allowed, preferably when they have been made in the water-based decaffeination process. Caffeine stimulates insulin production, causing your blood sugar to rise and then crash. If you're vulnerable to unstable blood sugar, this could mean fatigue, irritability, and cravings for carbohydrates. Try eliminating caffeine from your diet for a couple of weeks and see how you feel. If you notice that your energy levels even out, caffeine definitely affects your blood sugar and should be avoided.

As I explained back in Chapter 11, tea is an excellent source of antioxidant flavonoids, particularly the phenols that, among other benefits, help prevent cancer. The antioxidant capacity of an eight-ounce cup of freshly brewed green tea is anywhere from four to five times as great as a serving of kale; for black tea, the kind found in most tea bags, the antioxidant capacity is almost as high.

I strongly recommend at least one cup of freshly brewed tea a day as part of your antiaging diet; in fact, I recommend two cups a day of green tea. Make the tea using pure water and sweeten it if you wish only with noncaloric sweeteners like saccharin, stevia, or sucralose. Most important, do not add milk or cream to your tea. The proteins in the milk will bind with the phenols in the tea and make the phenols hard to absorb.

A recent study from Scotland illustrates my point— and also shows how misleading epidemiological studies can be. Researchers found that people who drank coffee had reduced levels of heart disease, while tea drinking was linked to higher levels, despite tea's much higher antioxidant content. The researchers attributed the difference to the fact that coffee drinkers were younger, were more affluent, and led healthier lives in general. What was never discussed in the study, however, is the fact that tea drinkers in Scotland usually add milk or cream and at least one teaspoon of sugar to each cup of tea—additives that would negate the benefits.[1] We know from other community health studies, such as the well-known Zutphen study of Dutch men, that tea drinking has definite beneficial effects on your cardiovascular health, as well as helping to prevent strokes and cancer.

What about alcoholic beverages? Several studies have shown that having a drink a day, especially a glass of red wine, has a beneficial effect on the heart. If you're already in the habit of having a daily cocktail or glass of wine with dinner, and if your weight is normal and you have no blood sugar instability, then by all means continue to have your daily drink. Those are a lot of ifs, and I find that nearly half of my patients should not be drinking alcohol at all. But when you do drink alcohol, stick to dry wine or straight liquor with a sugarless mixer like seltzer or diet soda. Avoid beer and dessert wines.

HOW MUCH SHOULD I EAT?

Perhaps you've been wondering, as you've been reading along in this chapter, exactly what amount constitutes a "serving." After all, other diet books tell you exactly how much of each food to eat, down to the last ounce. Those of you who have read my earlier books already know that I take the opposite approach. Counting calories and portions has very little to do with a diet that will help you live to a ripe old age—that is, as long as you remain at your ideal weight.

My general rule is to eat the amount that makes you feel comfortable. Whatever that quantity is, it's the amount that fills you up and satisfies you with a variety of delicious foods. You'll find that by cutting the simple carbohydrates out of your diet and substituting protein, fats, and complex carbohydrates, your appetite will be quickly satisfied without even having to think about calories, much less count them. Overeating becomes almost impossible.

How often you eat is just as important as what you eat. Try to start each day with a large, high-protein breakfast—a cheese omelette, for example. Eating at least three full meals a day is essential for keeping your blood sugar steady. As a variation, many of my patients find they actually do better on four to six smaller meals a day, including a protein snack before bed. Remember, the quality of your food is what counts, not the quantity.

So what exactly is *your* food, the food that's precisely right for helping you defy age and live a long and healthy life? We'll find that out next.

21

LIVING THE AGE-DEFYING DIET

Let's start this chapter with a pop quiz. How much sugar does the average American eat each day? I think you'll be amazed by the answer: twenty teaspoons. That's twenty of those little sugar packets, or nearly seven ounces, or almost a cup. Since 1983, sugar consumption in this country has increased 28 percent. In the form of table sugar, high-fructose corn syrup, or other caloric sweeteners, sugar now accounts for 16 percent of the total calories consumed by the average American. Even worse, sugar is now 20 percent of teenagers' calories.[1]

Here's another question. How many adult Americans are overweight? The answer: some 97 million people, or 55 percent of the population.[2]

Could there possibly be any connection? Not if you ask the U.S. Department of Agriculture, the people who bring you the infamous food pyramid. According to them, ten teaspoons of sugar a day are just fine. I wonder if that is what is meant by the advice in the food pyramid to use sugar "sparingly."

In this chapter, I'm going to teach you how to throw the food pyramid out the window and select the foods you should eat for a long and healthy life. The very first food you're going to throw out the window is sugar, followed immediately by the refined carbohydrates that are the basis of the food pyramid. Instead of these foods, we'll look at the foods you should be eating to help you defy and/or counter the effects of aging—exactly which vegetables and fruits are ideal for your personal age-defying diet program.

YOUR IDEAL CARBOHYDRATE LEVEL

We've said over and over again in this book that it's important to keep your carbohydrate consumption low. Okay, how low? Since one diet does not fit all, you now need to discover the answer to that for yourself. Simply put, you need to figure out the most generous level of carbohydrate consumption that both corresponds to your own individual metabolism and keeps you at your normal weight.

Although it's less than likely, given the statistics about Americans and excess weight, I'll start with the assumption that you are of normal weight, or even underweight, or have achieved normal weight through successful dieting. This allows me to teach you how to differentiate those carbohydrates most likely to make you healthier from those that have been creating epidemics of diabetes, heart disease, and shortened life spans.

Those of you with a weight problem, even if it is under control through dieting, have even greater need of this information, because in order both to achieve your ideal weight and stay there, you will have to find the nutritional elements of healthy carbohydrates from a relatively low number of total carbohydrates.

The first and most essential step in dealing with your carbohydrate intake is to obtain an accurate estimate of what your total daily allowance of carbohydrates should be. In *Dr. Atkins' New Diet Revolution*, which I urge overweight readers to read and follow, I taught that there are two levels of daily carbohydrate intake that must be identified for each individual. One applies only to overweight people; I gave it the name Critical Carbohydrate Level for Losing (CCLL). This is the number of daily grams of carbohydrate intake below which there is automatic weight loss. The other level applies to everyone. I gave it the name Critical Carbohydrate Level for Maintenance (CCLM). This is the carbohydrate intake level above which you will gain weight.

To expand this concept as a guideline for everyone, I must add to it the concepts of blood sugar stabilization and glycosylation as pro-aging abnormalities (refer back to Chapter 19 for more on these concepts). Further, for those few of you who simply do not gain weight, I must change the term to read Ideal Carbohydrate Level for Maintenance (ICLM), because your goal is health preservation, not weight control.

If you have a weight-gaining tendency, your personal CCLM could be anywhere from 25 to 90 grams of carbohydrates a day. How can you know what your daily carbohydrate intake should be within that fairly broad range? Well, every person is different, but if you've already lost weight on my low-carbohydrate diet, you have a good idea of what the right level is for you, based on what you had to do to lose weight. Your CCLM will only be around 10 grams higher than your level for losing slowly.

If you had high metabolic resistance and needed to restrict your carbohydrate intake to 15 grams or less, your CCLM will be even lower, probably between 25 and 40 grams a day. People with moderate metabolic resistance will probably end up with a carbohydrate intake between 40 and 60 grams a day. People with low metabolic resistance will probably find that between 60 and 90 carbohydrate grams a day is good for them.

But even if you've never had a weight problem, you're not off the carbohydrate hook. To defy the aging process, you must still keep your carbohydrates to the lowest amount consistent with feeling your best. For you, that may add as much as 90 grams to 150 grams a day. Remember, your goal here is not weight loss, it's the prevention of health problems related to aging. Most of those problems are related to excess carbohydrate consumption, even among people of normal weight.

These gram counts are simply guidelines, however. If your weight starts to creep up when you're taking in 60 grams of carbohydrates a day, then clearly you must cut back to the level that keeps your weight steady. Conversely, if you start to lose weight on 60 grams a day, it's an opportunity to add one or two servings of health-providing carbohydrates each day.

The main reason I have suggested keeping carbohydrate intake low, even without a weight problem, is the fact that stable blood sugar is very important to defying aging. And for that, you simply need to restrict your intake of carbohydrates, especially refined carbohydrates.

BALANCING CARBOHYDRATES

The foods you eat in the age-defying diet should be selected on the basis of two criteria: They should be low in carbohydrates and high in antioxidants. It is crucial to balance the two. Fortunately, many of the best low-carbohydrate foods are also very high in artery-protecting, cancer-fighting antioxidants, such as carotenoids.

Of course, we have long known how to measure carbohydrates; now, we also know how to measure antioxidant level. Some recent studies have used a sophisticated assay technique that can accurately measure the total antioxidant capacity of foods,[3] so we now have the tools to analyze exactly which vegetables and fruits best represent the combination of being low in carbs and high in antioxidants.

The pioneering effort to measure antioxidant level began at the Jean Mayer USDA Human Nutrition Center on Aging at Tufts University. It is indeed heartening that the Department of Agriculture is involved in this effort; it offers hope that our own government will eventually come to realize the folly of the food pyramid and recognize that significant work done by its own scientists points in another, much healthier direction.

At the Atkins Center, we have taken this extremely important research a step further. By looking at both the antioxidant scores of common vegetables and fruits *and* at their carbohydrate content, we have been able to determine the ratio of antioxidant value to carbohydrate grams. The higher the ratio, the more antioxidant protection you get per gram of carbohydrate. With these ratios, you now have a scientifically accurate way to choose the foods that are best for you.

Let's start with vegetables. Table 21.1 ranks popular vegetables in descending order of antioxidant protection and gives their antioxidant score. (The score is based on a complex formula that compares the antioxidant capacity of the vegetable to a standard called the Trolox equivalent.) The table also lists the carbohydrate content of a typical serving of the vegetable and gives you the antioxidant/carbohydrate ratio.

As you can see, you get the most antioxidant protection per typical serving from garlic and kale, and the least protection from celery and cucumbers. When you look at the antioxidant/carbohydrate ratio, however, you easily see that some foods that are high on the antioxidant scale are also high in carbohydrates; they therefore have a low ratio. Corn, for instance, is 7.2 on the antioxidant scale, but there are 20.6 grams of carbohydrate

Table 21.1

Total Antioxidant Capacity of Common Vegetables

VEGETABLE	ANTIOXIDANT SCORE (PER SERVING)*	CARBOHYDRATES (IN GRAMS)	A/C RATIO
Kale	24.1	3.7	6.5
Garlic (1 clove)	23.2	1.0	23.2
Spinach	17.0	3.4	5.0
Brussels sprouts	15.8	6.8	2.3
Broccoli	12.9	4.0	3.2
Beets	11.7	5.7	2.1
Red bell pepper (raw)	8.1	3.2	2.5
Corn	7.2	20.6	0.3
Onion (1 tablespoon)	5.6	0.9	6.2
Eggplant	5.1	3.2	1.6
Cauliflower	5.1	2.9	1.8
Cabbage	4.8	4.0	1.2
Potato (1 whole)	4.6	51.0	0.09
Sweet potato	4.3	27.7	0.15
Leaf lettuce (1 leaf)	4.1	0.5	8.2
Green beans	3.9	4.9	0.8
Carrots	3.4	8.2	0.4
Yellow squash	2.8	3.9	0.7
Iceberg lettuce (1 leaf)	2.3	0.4	5.8
Celery (raw)	1.1	0.75	1.5
Cucumber (raw)	1.1	1.5	0.7

*Servings are one-half cup cooked unless otherwise indicated.

SOURCES: Cao G., E. Sofic, and R. L. Prior. "Antioxidant Capacity of Tea and Common Vegetables." *Journal of Agricultural and Food Chemistry* 44 (1996): 3426–31; Pennington, Jean A. T., ed. *Bowes & Church's Food Values of Portions Commonly Used.* 16th ed. *Philadelphia: Lippincott 1994.*

in a half-cup serving. That makes the ratio of antioxidant protection to carbohydrates in corn a low 0.3.

In fact, overall, the starchier a vegetable is, the lower its ratio of antioxidant protection to carbohydrates. Sweet potatoes, for instance, are often touted as being particularly healthy because of their high beta-carotene content. In fact, as the table shows, sweet potatoes aren't particularly high in antioxidants relative to other vegetables. They are very high in carbohydrates, however; a typical baked sweet potato contains nearly 28 grams. That makes the antioxidant/carbohydrate ratio for a sweet potato only 0.15. If you're going to eat only 40 grams of carbohydrates a day, you should probably think twice about sweet potatoes; you'd be much better off using your carb allowance on foods that give you a higher carbohydrate/antioxidant ratio, such as greens, broccoli, red bell peppers, and so on.

You'll note that the table includes the scientifically established antioxidant values for only some twenty-one vegetables. Research in this area is still in the early stages, and only a small number of vegetables have been analyzed. Vegetables not on the list are not precluded from your age-defying diet, however; just avoid the starchy ones.

Variety in vegetables, as in anything, is good for you. For one thing, it keeps you from becoming bored by your food. You also avoid the possibility of developing food sensitivities, which typically arise when people eat the same few foods day in and day out.

FAVORITE FRUITS

The same analytical techniques applied to vegetables have been applied to a variety of fruits. The results tell us exactly which fruits have the highest antioxidant/carbohydrate ratio, as listed in Table 21.2.

As with the vegetables, the fruits that are highest in antioxidant protection turn out to be the ones that are also lowest in carbohydrates. Blueberries, the top antioxidant fruit with a ranking of 24, have only 10.3 grams of carbohydrate in a half cup; they thus have a winning carbohydrate/antioxidant ratio of 2.3. Compare that to a banana, which has 13.4 grams of carbohydrate and an antioxidant ranking of just 2.1. Its ratio is 0.2. It's pretty

Table 21.2

Total Antioxidant Capacity of Common Fruits			
FRUIT	ANTIOXIDANT SCORE (PER SERVING)*	CARBOHYDRATES (IN GRAMS)	A/C RATIO
Blueberries	24.0	10.3	2.3
Blackberries	20.0	9.2	2.2
Strawberries	12.4	5.3	2.3
Plum	8.4	8.6	1.0
Orange	6.8	8.2	0.8
Kiwi	5.5	11.3	0.5
Pink grapefruit	4.5	9.5	0.5
Red grapes	3.9	7.9	0.5
Green grapes	2.9	7.9	0.4
Banana	2.1	13.4	0.2
Apple	1.9	10.5	0.2
Tomato	1.6	2.9	0.5
Pear	1.2	12.5	0.1
Honeydew melon	0.9	7.8	0.1

*Serving is one-half cup raw.

SOURCES: Wang, H., G. Cao, and R. L. Prior. "Total Antioxidant Capacity of Fruits." *Journal of Agricultural and Food Chemistry* 44 (1996): 701–05; Prior, R. L. et al. "Antioxidant Capacity as influenced by Total Phenolic and Anthocyanin Content, Maturity, and Variety of Vaccinium Species." *Journal of Agricultural and Food Chemistry* 46 (1998): 2686–93; Pennington, Jean A. T., ed. *Bowes & Church's Food Values of Portions Commonly Used.* 16th ed. Philadelphia: Lippincott, 1994.

obvious that blueberries are by far the better choice.

In fact, berries of any kind are an excellent choice. A dish of blueberries or strawberries, topped with whipped cream or mixed with ricotta cheese sweetened with stevia or sucralose, is one of my favorite desserts. One word of caution: Frozen berries are almost as high in antioxidants as fresh, but they may have added sugar. Read the label carefully and choose a brand that has no added sugar.

In addition to berries, other good low-sugar fruit choices are apricots, cherries, grapes, peaches, and plums. Melons such as honeydew and cantaloupe are also excellent choices. Don't forget that technically speaking, avocados and tomatoes are fruits. Avocados are an excellent source of monounsaturated fat; try to find California avocados, which are much lower in carbohydrates than Florida avocados (12 grams to 27).

You might think that if a fruit is a good source of antioxidants, then fruit juice, which is more concentrated, would be better. That's only partially true. In the case of commercial grape juice, which is made using dark-skinned purple grapes, the antioxidant level is indeed higher, mostly because the purple Concord grapes used in the juice have more flavonoids. Tomato juice also has a higher antioxidant score than fresh tomatoes. Orange juice and apple juice, however, have much lower antioxidant scores than the fresh fruit.

Overall, avoid fruit juices. They are highly concentrated sources of sugar, both naturally and often from added sugar as well. Commercial grape juices, even the so-called organic brands, often are either mixed with apple juice or contain added high-fructose corn syrup as a sweetener. And since the juices don't have the fruit's fiber, which slows the sugar's entry into your bloodstream, fruit juices will send your blood sugar on a roller-coaster ride.

If you crave something sweet for dessert or a snack, fruit is certainly a better choice than a candy bar or cookies. The lower glycemic index of some fruits means that your blood sugar stays steadier. Even so, sugar is sugar and should be kept to a minimum, so select the lower-carbohydrate fruits whenever possible.

Watch out for the higher-carb fruits like apples, bananas, nectarines, oranges, and pears. Dried fruits such as raisins, dates, figs, and prunes are extremely high in sugar and should be avoided. Also avoid any sort of canned fruits, especially the ones in heavy syrup.

Relatively speaking, vegetables have more antioxidant value per carbohydrate gram than fruits. Even so, I suggest that if your ICLM is not especially low, you use some of your daily carbohydrate ration to eat one or two cups of fruit a day. We have yet to identify all the valuable phytochemicals, or even all the antioxidants in foods, so it makes sense to eat as wide a variety of fresh fruits and vegetables as possible to give yourself the maximum protection.

COUNTING CAROTENOIDS

I've already discussed the incredible importance of carotenoids such as beta-carotene and lycopene for your health (check back to Chapter 10 for details). Here I'm going to get specific about the carotenoid content of common fruits and vegetables. Table 21.3 lists the top nineteen carotenoid foods and gives the ratio of carotenoids to carbohydrates.

The best sources of carotenoids in foods are dark green leafy vegetables and orange-colored foods like carrots. As you can see from the table, the high carbohydrate content of carrots is outweighed here by their very high carotenoid content—the carotenoid/carbohydrate ratio is 11.3. But collard greens are an even better choice, with a carotenoid/carbohydrate ratio of 32.4. For just about half the carbohydrates of carrots, collard greens give you nearly three times the antioxidant pro-

Table 21.3

Carotenoids in Fruits and Vegetables			
FOOD	CAROTENOID CONTENT (IN MCG PER G)	CARBOHYDRATES (IN GRAMS)	C/C RATIO
Kale	220.0	3.7	59.5
Turnip greens	130.2	1.6	81.4
Collards	126.2	3.9	32.4
Spinach	122.9	3.4	36.1
Sweet potato	94.8	27.7	3.4
Carrots	92.5	8.2	11.3
Butternut squash	57.0	10.7	5.3
Red bell pepper (raw)	46.4	3.2	14.5
Swiss chard	40.0	3.6	11.1
Romaine lettuce (raw)	39.1	0.7	55.8
Tomato (raw)	36.6	2.9	12.6
Broccoli	32.7	4.0	8.2
Apricots (raw)	25.5	7.9	3.2
Zucchini	25.4	3.5	7.3
Brussels sprouts	20.5	6.8	3.0
Cantaloupe (raw)	16.6	6.7	2.5
Green beans	13.4	4.9	2.7
Endive (raw)	9.6	0.8	12.0
Corn	9.5	20.6	0.5

NOTES: Carotenoid figures are total carotenoid content, including alpha-carotene, beta-carotene, lutein, zeaxanthin, lycopene. Portions are one-half cup cooked unless noted otherwise.

SOURCE: USDA-NCC Carotenoid Database for U.S. Foods, 1998: Pennington, Jean A. T., ed. *Bowes & Church's Food Values of Portions Commonly Used.* 16th ed. Philadelphia: Lippincott, 1994.

tections. Which will you choose? I think the answer is pretty obvious.

Cooking high-carotenoid foods actually increases their nutritional value by breaking down the tough cell walls and releasing the carotenoids, especially beta-carotene. To preserve the other nutrients, however, cook vegetables gently by steaming them in as little water as possible or by sautéing them lightly in olive oil or butter.

By the same token, the processing of tomatoes, the best source of the carotenoid lycopene, is what actually releases the lycopene, a superb cancer preventive, particularly of prostate cancer. That means that tomato juice or puree has considerably more lycopene than an uncooked tomato. In addition, lycopene is best absorbed by your body if the tomatoes are eaten with some dietary fat, such as olive oil. Table 21.4 lists the best sources for lycopene in foods and gives the ratio of lycopene content to carbohydrates for each. Stay away from to-

Table 21.4

The Lycopene Content of Foods				
FOOD	SERVING SIZE	LYCOPENE	CARBOHYDRATES	L/C
Tomato puree	1 cup	35.6	25.1	1.4
Tomato juice	1 cup	25.0	10.3	2.4
Watermelon	1 medium slice	14.7	11.5	1.3
Tomato paste	2 tablespoons	13.8	6.2	2.2
Tomato soup, condensed	1 cup	9.7	22.4	0.4
Pink grapefruit	one half	4.9	9.5	0.5
Tomato, raw	1 medium	3.7	5.7	0.6
Tomato ketchup	1 tablespoon	2.7	4.1	0.7

SOURCES: USDA—NCC Carotenoid Database for U.S. Foods. 1998: Pennington, Jean A. T., ed. *Bowes & Church's Food Values of Portions Commonly Used*, 16th ed. Philadelphia: Lippincott, 1994.

mato ketchup—it's approximately one-third sugar. In fact, all tomato foods are high in carbohydrates. Eight ounces of tomato juice, for example, contain about 10 grams. You may want to take lycopene supplements instead.

Lutein and zeaxanthin, carotenoids found in vegetables and eggs, are crucial for protecting your eyesight from age-related macular degeneration. (Check back to Chapter 10 for more on this.) Because the two nutrients are hard to break out in analysis, and because you need them both, Table 21.5 lists the top lutein/zeaxanthin

Table 21.5

Lutein and Zeaxanthin Content of Foods			
FOOD	LUTEIN/ ZEAXANTHIN (IN MCG PER G)	CARBOHYDRATES (IN GRAMS)	LZ/C RATIO
Kale	158.0	3.7	42.7
Turnip greens	84.4	1.6	52.7
Collard greens	80.9	3.9	20.7
Spinach	70.4	3.4	20.7
Romaine lettuce (raw)	26.3	0.7	37.6
Broccoli	22.3	4.0	5.6
Zucchini	21.2	3.5	6.1
Corn	18.0	20.6	0.9
Peas	13.5	12.5	1.1
Brussels sprouts	12.9	6.8	1.9
Green beans	7.0	4.9	1.4
Okra	3.9	5.8	0.7
Orange (raw)	1.8	8.2	0.2
Tomato (raw)	1.3	2.9	7.1
Peach (raw)	0.6	4.9	0.1

NOTE: Portions are one-half cup cooked unless otherwise noted.

SOURCE: USDA-NCC Carotenoid Database for U.S. Foods, 1998 and Jean A. T., Pennington, ed. *Bowes & Church's Food Values of Portions Commonly Used*, 16th ed. (Philadelphia: J. B. Lippincott Company, 1994).

foods and gives the lutein/zeaxanthin-to-carbohydrate ratio.

THE VALUE OF FRUITS AND VEGETABLES

A bedrock principle of alternative medicine is that diet plays a crucial role in health. As a complementary practitioner, I know from my own experience with thousands of patients and from avidly reading numerous studies from Europe and the United States that those who consume a diet rich in fresh fruits and vegetables have significantly better health profile than those who eat other carbohydrates. (No study to date, however, has compared them to an extremely low total carbohydrate intake.)

For example, a 1996 meta-analysis looked at well over two hundred studies that had been done on the relationship between vegetable and fruit consumption and the risk of cancer. The impressive conclusion: There is strong evidence for a protective effect against cancer from these foods.[4]

An interesting recent study compared cardiac risk factors in men from Czechoslovakia, where the death rate from coronary heart disease is high, to the risk factors for men in Germany, where the coronary death rate is moderate, and in Israel, where the coronary death rate is low. Most of the traditional indicators, such as cholesterol, were about the same for all three groups. The Czech men, however, had very low levels of carotenoids compared to the Israeli men. The average Czech man had a beta-carotene level of 60 mcg, while his Israeli counterpart had 102 mcg; for lycopene, the numbers were 84 mcg to 223 mcg. Why the difference? The Czech men ate very few fresh fruits and vegetables.[5]

Other researchers have recently studied precisely the extent to which eating fresh fruits and vegetables increases your antioxidant level. In one of the studies, thirty-six healthy people went on a two-week diet regimen controlled for ten or more portions a day of fresh fruits and vegetables. Blood tests showed that the diet significantly increased the total antioxidant capacity of their blood.[6] A study of elderly women showed that their antioxidant levels were increased when they consumed strawberries, spinach, red wine, or vitamin C. Four hours later, their blood antioxidant levels had jumped by anywhere from 7 to 25 percent from the foods.[7]

I must point out that the comparison groups for every one of these studies were eating diets loaded with refined carbohydrates and that none were truly carbohydrate-restricted. The question thus remains: Do these studies prove that fruits and vegetables are good for you? Or is it more that refined "junk" carbohydrates are bad? Whatever the answer, I believe we can all benefit from eating the valuable carbohydrates and eliminating the junk.

THE WHOLE (GRAIN) STORY

One of the unfounded accusations that's often leveled against the Atkins Diet is that it forbids carbohydrates like bread, pasta, rice, and beans, to say nothing of the fruits and vegetables. During the induction phase of my weight loss diet, that's true—such carbohydrates are indeed prohibited. Once you reach your maintenance weight and have determined what your CCLM is, these foods can come back into your life to a limited extent. Let me stress again, however, that the more carbohydrates you eat, the faster you will age.

Make the most of the carbohydrates in your diet by eating unrefined whole grains whenever possible. Bread made with genuine whole wheat—not the brown-colored stuff that passes for whole wheat in most commercial breads—has more gourmet appeal than the enriched white-flour variation. It's somewhat lower in carbohydrates than commercial bread and considerably more satisfying. Because the whole grains still have their bran, which is the outer coating on the grain, the bread has a lower glycemic index and much more nutrition, including all the crucial B vitamins.

One problem with whole grains is that they contain phytic acid, the same substance that is present in high levels in the skins of beans. In your intestines, phytic acid combines with zinc, calcium, magnesium, and iron to form phytates. The phytates are insoluble, so they pass out of your body, carrying the minerals with them. Over the long run, eating a diet high in whole grains, as many vegetarians and vegans do, can lead to outright mineral deficiency.

The phytic acid in whole grains and beans can be almost eliminated quite easily, however, with proper advance preparation. In the case of whole wheat, for example, natural fermentation removes most of the phytic acid, as is done with sourdough breads. An alternative to whole-wheat bread is bread made from sprouted grains—the sprouting process removes much of the phytic acid.

Another way to reduce the phytic acid in whole grains is to soak them for several hours in buttermilk. The lactic acid in the buttermilk breaks down the phytic acid in the bran. This is similar to what you do when you soak uncooked beans in water for several hours before cooking; the soaking and rinsing remove most of the phytic acid from the skins and also improve digestibility.*

At the Atkins Center, we often find that food allergies underlie numerous chronic health problems. Many of our patients turn out to be sensitive to the gluten in wheat and in such other grains as rye, barley, and oats. I attribute the dramatic improvement in these patients to the elimination of gluten grains from their diet—although we improve their nutrition in a variety of other ways as well.

The easiest way to find out if gluten is a problem for you is simply to stay away from foods that contain gluten grains for a while. That's certainly not a hardship if you're following the age-defying diet. If your ICLM allows you to have more carbohydrates in your diet, substitute beans, brown rice, millet, and other gluten-free grains.

Unrefined whole grains are generally a little lower in carbohydrates than their refined counterparts. One cup of cooked brown rice, for instance, has about 45 grams, whereas the same amount of white rice has 57 grams. You probably won't find many high-quality whole-grain products in your supermarket. In my experience, even well-stocked health food stores carry a lot of products that claim to be made from whole grains but really aren't. Read the ingredients labels carefully when you buy products like whole-wheat pasta or buckwheat noodles.

The fact is, however, that the human digestive tract is simply not well designed for digesting grains. The proteins in grain, especially the gluten, are very difficult to digest, even if you don't have apparent gluten prob-

---

*An excellent cookbook with many recipes for cooking with whole foods is *Nourishing Traditions* by Sally Fallon (San Diego: Promotion Publishing, 1995).

lems. Too much grain, especially of the highly refined kind, is behind many of the cases of food allergies, irritable bowel, chronic indigestion, and yeast overgrowth that I see every day. I much prefer to see my patients who are eligible for more carbohydrates add potatoes, yams, succotash, and lentils instead of grains to their diet.

Beans and legumes, such as kidney beans, chickpeas, and lentils, are fairly high in carbohydrates, but I feel their high vegetable protein content, high fiber content, and beneficial vitanutrient content make them a good addition to an age-defying diet. When properly soaked for several hours before cooking to remove phytic acid from the skins, beans are also quite easy to digest. They are also very filling—just half a cup is a substantial portion that generally contains between 20 and 30 grams of carbohydrates.

What's the lesson? Once you've determined your appropriate carbohydrate level, get your carb intake in a variety of fresh vegetables plus fresh fruits in smaller amounts. The broad array of antioxidants found in these foods is much more effective at protecting you from free radical damage than any one supplemental vitanutrient can be. Nevertheless, vitanutrient supplements are an important part of your age-defying diet, so let's explore exactly how you can make them part of your life.

SUGGESTED MENUS

The month's worth of menus that follow were designed to guide you in eating a diet rich in antioxidants—and one that offers the most age-defying punch. The meals provide a broad spectrum of antioxidants: vitamin C, lycopene, carotenoids, selenium, vitamin E, leutin, zeax-anthin, glutathione, and more. Eating and living the age-defying way is good for you and tastes great too.

MENUS AND RECIPES

The following menus are not meant to be followed to the letter or in this exact order. They offer an idea of the many healthful and enjoyable possibilities available to an age-defying dieter.

You may interchange any protein dishes—meat, fowl, seafood, and wild game—as well as the vegetables.

Use garlic, onions, leeks, shallots, and scallions as liberally as you can.

Refer to the Atkins Ratio for the best vegetable choices.

Use natural spices and herbs liberally. (Future research may prove them extremely valuable. Check our Web site for reports.)

You will find Atkins-approved diet alternatives available for your food planning. Check our Web site regularly.

Note: An asterisk after a dish means that a recipe is included.

MENUS

DAY 1
Breakfast
Cheese omelette with spinach and mushrooms
Bacon
Tomato juice

Lunch
Fennel salad with flank steak and nuts

Dinner
Roast leg of lamb
Cauliflower and Swiss chard sautéed in garlic and olive oil
Cucumber and red onion salad
Blueberries and cream

Day 2
Breakfast
Broccoli frittata
Grapefruit

Lunch
Chicken Caesar salad

Dinner
Grilled swordfish
Mashed turnips with garlic butter
Broccoli rabe sautéed in garlic and olive oil

DAY 3
Breakfast
Smoked salmon rolled around cream cheese
Scallion stalks
Fresh-squeezed tomato juice

Lunch
Chef salad with choice of meats and cheeses
Yeast-free high-fiber crisp breads

Dinner
Roast loin of pork
Broccoli
Baked sweet potato

DAY 4
Breakfast
Eggs Benedict with spinach (no English muffin)
Fresh-squeezed green vegetable juice

Lunch
Salmon burgers
Cauliflower pureed with Romano cheese and cream

Dinner
T-bone steak with sautéed mushrooms, onions, and garlic in olive oil
Green beans almandine
Strawberries and cream

DAY 5
Breakfast
Ricotta cheese with cinnamon, splenda, and walnuts
Fresh sausage links
Peach slices

Lunch
Pesto chicken salad on mesclun greens
Yeast-free high-fiber crisp breads

Dinner
Baked grouper with butter and garlic
Brussels sprouts sautéed in olive oil
Green salad

DAY 6
Breakfast
Fresh-baked ham slices rolled with Swiss cheese and spinach leaves
Mixed berries

Lunch
Blue cheese burger with bacon
Sweet potato french fries
Green salad

Dinner
Veal ribs
Sautéed kale with garlic and olive oil
Fresh buffalo mozzarella with tomato and basil
Strawberries dipped in low-carbohydrate chocolate mousse

DAY 7
Breakfast
Breakfast pizza*

Lunch
Turkey teriyaki with scallions, broccoli, snow peas, sesame oil, fresh ginger, soy sauce, and sesame seeds

Dinner
Baby back ribs
Baked sweet potato
Creamed spinach

DAY 8
Breakfast
Sardines with sour cream and fresh dill
Fresh-squeezed tomato juice

Lunch
Steak salad with olives, avocado, shallots, cheese, and dressing

Dinner
Onion soup with melted mozzarella
Roast turkey with gravy
Snow peas with butter

DAY 9
Breakfast
BLT with melted cheese
Honeydew melon

Lunch
Endive salad with diced ham, Roquefort cheese, scallions, and walnuts

Dinner
Spicy shrimp stir-fry with bok choy, carrots, snow peas, broccoli, celery, sesame oil, and sesame seeds

DAY 10
Breakfast
Fried eggs
Bacon
Yeast-free high-fiber crisp breads

Lunch
Asian beef salad*

Dinner
Lobster with garlic butter
Mixed grilled vegetables with garlic and olive oil

DAY 11
Breakfast
Pancakes made with low-carbohydrate bake mix, topped
with butter, low-carbohydrate syrup, strawberries, and
whipped cream
Sausage links

Lunch
Buffalo shish kebab with fresh vegetables
Turnip "fries"*

Dinner
Meat loaf
Kale sautéed in garlic and olive oil
Mashed turnips

DAY 12
Breakfast
Western omelette
Melon

Lunch
Crab salad stuffed in avocado
Rosemary-mushroom soup*

Dinner
Venison
Cabbage sautéed in garlic and butter
Stewed tomatoes

DAY 13
Breakfast
Egg, cheese, and bacon sandwich on low-carbohydrate toast
Peach

Lunch
Tofu, green beans, sun-dried tomatoes, and goat cheese*

Dinner
Roast lamb shoulder
Broccoli rabe sautéed in garlic and olive oil

DAY 14
Breakfast
Caviar and sour cream
Fresh-squeezed mixed vegetable juice

Lunch
Seafood salad on mesclun greens with olive oil and vinegar dressing

Dinner
Roasted stuffed Cornish hen*
Broccoli
Green salad

DAY 15
Breakfast
California breakfast burrito*

Lunch
Spinach salad with grilled chicken, shallots, hard-boiled eggs, bacon, fresh blue cheese

Dinner
Orange ginger tofu stir-fry, with tofu, red pepper, cauliflower, broccoli, carrots, fresh ginger, and grated orange peel

DAY 16
Breakfast
Wild mushroom and Gruyere cheese omelette

Lunch
Mediterranean salad, with mixed greens, mozzarella, prosciutto, sun-dried tomatoes, green pepper, olives, and garlic, with olive oil and vinegar dressing

Dinner
Chicken parmigiana topped with grilled eggplant and fresh tomato sauce

DAY 17
Breakfast
Chopped whitefish salad
Canadian bacon
Cantaloupe

Lunch
Reuben sandwich in low-carbohydrate tortilla
Pork rinds

Dinner
Roast duck
Grilled eggplant
Spaghetti squash with fresh tomato sauce

DAY 18
Breakfast
Cheese pancakes with blackberries

Lunch
Asian beef salad*

Dinner
Red snapper en papillote*
Corn on the cob
Green salad

DAY 19
Scrambled eggs with mixed vegetables
Fresh sausage links
Fresh-squeezed tomato juice

Lunch
Burgundy beef stew*

Dinner
Grilled grouper over celery, leeks, bok choy, and lemon

DAY 20
Breakfast
Poached eggs with Canadian bacon and hollandaise sauce
Melon

Lunch
Trio salad of chicken, shrimp, and tuna on arugula

Dinner
Beef tenderloin and greens Dijon*

DAY 21
Breakfast
Fried green tomatoes*

Lunch
Chunky chili chicken*

Dinner
Grilled tuna steak with wasabi and mayonnaise
Roasted bulb of garlic with low-carbohydrate bread
Grilled yellow squash

DAY 22
Breakfast
Blueberry scones*
Cottage cheese

Lunch
Chicken salad with dandelion greens, mustard greens, chicory, feta cheese, and soy nuts in a low-cho dressing

Dinner
Baked salmon
Grilled portobello mushrooms and tomatoes with fresh cilantro

DAY 23
Breakfast
Low-carbohydrate shake with cream and blueberries
Deviled eggs

Lunch
Jamaican jerked beef*
Snow peas sautéed in garlic and olive oil

Dinner
Broiled pork chops
Butternut squash with garlic butter
Asparagus and cheese sauce

DAY 24
Breakfast
Fried eggs with corned beef hash*
Plum

Lunch
Turkey drumstick
Collard greens and scallions sautéed in garlic and butter

Dinner
Chicken cacciatore*
Brussels sprouts

DAY 25
Breakfast
Pineapple ricotta pancakes*

Lunch
Chicken fajitas with mixed vegetables, sour cream, and guacamole

Dinner
Shish kebabs with any meat or fish and choice of vegetables
Baked ratatouille*

DAY 26
Breakfast
Scrambled eggs with cheese, tomato, scallions, and mushrooms
Mixed berries with cream

Lunch
Cajun chicken with okra*

Dinner
Filet mignon
Mashed turnips with garlic butter
Julienne carrots

DAY 27
Breakfast
Cereal mix with fresh cranberries and cream

Lunch
Asparagus and leek soup*
Rotisserie chicken

Dinner
Thai beef grill*

DAY 28
Breakfast
Cottage cheese with mixed berries and nuts
Smoked sausage

Lunch
Sloppy Joe with ground beef, veal, or pork, sugarless
tomato paste, bell pepper, and onion, topped with melted
mozzarella
Yeast-free high-fiber crisp breads

Dinner
Broiled chicken with oregano, lemon, and capers
Buttered zucchini

RECIPES

BREAKFAST PIZZA

1½ cups low-carbohydrate bread machine mix
1 tablespoon plus 1½ teaspoons dough relaxer
1 teaspoon active dry yeast
3 tablespoons olive oil
6 tablespoons water
½ cup low-carbohydrate marinara sauce
½ cup grated cheese

1. Preheat the oven to 400°. In a bowl, whisk together
the bread mix, dough relaxer, and yeast. Stir in the olive
oil and water, 1 tablespoon at a time, until the dough

holds together. Knead for 3 to 5 minutes, until smooth.
2. Form the dough into a rectangle. Roll it out on a
cookie sheet to ¼ inch thick and about 8 by 10 inches.
Crimp the edge. Spread the marinara sauce and sprinkle
cheese evenly over the dough.
3. Bake for 15 minutes until crisp on the bottom. Slice
in quarters.

SERVES 4.

Asian Beef Salad

Marinade and Dressing:
3 cloves garlic, minced
4 green onions, chopped
¼ cup soy sauce
2 tablespoons olive oil
2 tablespoons rice wine vinegar
2 teaspoons sesame oil
¼ teaspoon curry powder
¼ teaspoon dried ginger

1½ pounds beef sirloin steak, cut cross-grain into
⅛-inch strips
6 cups mixed salad greens
1 red bell pepper, thinly sliced
8 ounces (1 can) water chestnuts, drained

1. Mix the marinade ingredients in a bowl. Pour half
into a resealable plastic bag. Add the steak and let it
stand in the refrigerator for at least 3 hours. Reserve the
rest of the marinade.
2. Grill or sauté the steak. Mix it with the salad greens,

bell pepper, and water chestnuts. Add the remaining dressing.

SERVES 4.

TURNIP "FRIES"

4 turnips, trimmed and peeled
1 tablespoon peanut or olive oil
salt

1. Place an oven rack in the upper third of the oven. Preheat the oven to 425°.
2. Slice the turnips in half-inch strips. Place them on a nonstick cookie sheet and drizzle with the oil. Toss the turnips until coated. Spread the turnip slices into a single layer and sprinkle them with salt.
3. Bake the fries, turning them several times, until browned and tender, about 30 minutes. Serve immediately.

SERVES 4.

ROSEMARY-MUSHROOM SOUP

3 tablespoons rosemary-garlic ghee
1 medium onion, chopped
2 cloves garlic
20 ounces mushrooms, sliced
2 tablespoons low-carbohydrate bake mix
1 can (14½ ounces) chicken broth plus 1½ cans water

1 teaspoon chopped fresh rosemary, or ½ teaspoon dried
salt and pepper
sour cream, optional

1. Heat the ghee in a large saucepan over medium heat.
Sauté the onion for 10 minutes, until golden. Add the
garlic and cook 1 minute more. Add the mushrooms and
cook 8 minutes, until soft. Add the bake mix and stir
until it is dissolved.
2. Gradually add the broth, water, and rosemary. Bring
to a boil, then reduce heat and simmer for 10 minutes.
Let the soup cool slightly. Puree half the soup in a
blender and return it to the saucepan. Season to taste
with salt and pepper. Garnish with a sprig of fresh rosemary and a swirl of sour cream, if desired.

SERVES 6.

GREEN BEANS, SUN-DRIED TOMATOES, AND GOAT CHEESE

1 pound green beans, trimmed and cut into 1-inch pieces
2 tablespoons extra-virgin olive oil
½ cup leeks, thinly sliced
2 cloves garlic, minced
½ cup white wine
2 tablespoons oil-packed sun-dried tomatoes, drained
and coarsely chopped
2 teaspoons chopped fresh thyme, or 1 teaspoon dried
salt and pepper
4 ounces soft goat cheese, crumbled

1. In a large, deep skillet, bring salted water to a boil.
Add the green beans and cook until crisp, about 5

minutes. Drain and rinse with cold water until cool.

2. In the same skillet, heat the olive oil over medium-high heat. Add the leeks and garlic and sauté until softened, about 3 minutes. Add the wine, tomatoes, and thyme and heat to boiling. Boil 1 minute and add the green beans. Heat. Add salt and pepper to taste.

3. Stir in the goat cheese and heat. Serve immediately.

SERVES 4.

ROASTED STUFFED CORNISH HENS

4 Cornish game hens
salt and pepper
¼ pound spicy pork sausage, casing removed
3 tablespoons butter
2 shallots, finely chopped
⅔ cup sliced mushrooms
2 ounces cream cheese
3 low-cho high-fiber crisps, crumbled
½ cup reduced-sodium chicken broth mixed with ½ cup water

1. Heat the oven to 375°. Set a rack in a large roasting pan. Rinse and pat dry the hens. Sprinkle inside and outside with salt and pepper.

2. In a medium saucepan over medium heat, brown the sausage. Drain the sausage on paper towels and wipe the saucepan. Melt 1 tablespoon of the butter and sauté the shallots until translucent, about 5 minutes. Add the mushrooms and cook 5 minutes more. Cool slightly, then return the sausage to the pan. Add the cream cheese and crackers and mix well.

3. Divide the stuffing among the hens. Tie the legs to-

gether with kitchen string. Arrange the hens on the rack. Melt the remaining butter and brush it over the hens. Roast for 20 to 25 minutes. Pour half the broth-water mixture on the bottom of the roasting pan. Roast another 20 to 25 minutes, or until the stuffing temperature is 180° on an instant thermometer.

4. Remove the birds from the rack. Skim off the fat from the pan and pour in the remaining broth mixture. On the stove top, cook over medium heat for 5 minutes, stirring, until the sauce thickens.

SERVES 4.

CALIFORNIA BREAKFAST BURRITOS

4 low-carbohydrate flour tortillas
1 tablespoon canola oil
½ green onion, chopped
4 ounces green chilies, chopped
1 tomato, peeled, seeded, and diced
¼ teaspoon salt
¼ teaspoon pepper
6 large eggs
pinch cayenne pepper
2 tablespoons chopped cilantro
¼ cup salsa
½ cup grated cheddar cheese

1. Heat the oven to 325°. Wrap the tortillas in foil and heat in the oven for 5 to 10 minutes.
2. Meanwhile, heat the oil in a nonstick skillet over medium-high heat. Add the onions, chilies, tomato, salt, and pepper and sauté 3 minutes. Push the mixture to the side of the pan.

3. In a small bowl, beat the eggs and the cayenne pepper. Add to the skillet and cook for 1 to 2 minutes, stirring, until it forms soft, creamy curds. Stir the vegetable mixture into the eggs.

4. Divide the mixture among the warm tortillas. Sprinkle each with cilantro, 1 tablespoon of the salsa, and 2 tablespoons of the cheese. Roll the tortillas into logs.

SERVES 4.

RED SNAPPER EN PAPILLOTE

1 small red pepper, cut into strips
4 green onions, cut into 2-inch strips
2 tablespoons chopped sun-dried tomatoes
4 red snapper fillets, about 8 ounces each
½ teaspoon dried oregano
½ teaspoon dried basil
salt and pepper
4 tablespoons olive oil

1. Heat the oven to 400°. Cut four 12-inch by 12-inch squares of foil. Fold each square in half, then open again. Mix the red pepper, onions, and sun-dried tomatoes in a bowl. Place one-quarter of the vegetable mixture on each foil square, about 1 inch from the fold.

2. Sprinkle the fish with the oregano, basil, salt, and pepper. Place one fillet on top of each vegetable mound. Drizzle with the olive oil. Seal and crimp the edges to make airtight packets. (The fish packets can be made several hours ahead of time and refrigerated.)

3. Place the packets on a cookie sheet and bake for 15 minutes. Open the packets directly on dinner plates.

SERVES 4.

BURGUNDY BEEF STEW

½ cup low-carbohydrate bake mix
3 pounds beef chuck or round, cut into cubes
¼ pound sliced bacon
1 tablespoon oil
1 medium onion, chopped
1 carrot, chopped
1 celery stalk, chopped
2 cloves garlic, minced
2 cups dry red wine
1 can reduced-sodium beef broth, plus 1 can water
1 bay leaf
½ teaspoon dried thyme
1 tablespoon butter
½ pound button mushrooms

1. Spread the bake mix on a plate. Dredge the beef cubes in the bake mix and tap off the excess. In a large Dutch oven, sauté the bacon until crisp. Remove the bacon, and when it cools, crumble it and place it aside.
2. Add the oil to the bacon fat. Brown the beef in batches and transfer it to a platter. Add the onion, carrot, celery, and garlic to the Dutch oven and cook 8 minutes, until softened. Add the wine and increase the heat to high. Boil until the liquid is reduced to 1 cup, about 5 minutes.
3. Return the beef and accumulated juices to the Dutch oven. Add the beef broth and water, bay leaf, and thyme. Reduce the heat to low and simmer, partially covered, for 1½ hours, until the beef is tender.
4. Melt the butter in a skillet. Sauté the mushrooms over medium heat until golden, about 5 minutes. Add the

mushrooms and the reserved bacon to the stew. Remove the bay leaf.

SERVES 6.

BEEF TENDERLOIN AND GREENS DIJON

Dressing:
½ cup olive oil
¼ cup Dijon-style mustard
¼ cup balsamic vinegar
1 clove garlic, minced
½ packet sugar substitute
½ teaspoon dried basil
¼ teaspoon pepper

1½ pounds beef tenderloin tips
1 tablespoon olive oil
½ teaspoon salt
¼ teaspoon pepper
8-10 ounces mixed salad greens
Atkins croutons

1. Whisk together the dressing ingredients until creamy. Set aside.
2. Cut the beef tips into 1- to 1½-inch pieces. Heat the oil in a large nonstick skillet over medium-high heat. Add the beef in two batches and stir-fry for 2 to 3 minutes, until the outside is no longer pink. Remove from the skillet and season with salt and pepper.
3. Toss the salad greens with ½ cup of the dressing. Arrange the greens on a platter and top with beef and croutons. Serve with the remaining dressing on the side.

SERVES 4.

FRIED GREEN TOMATOES

4 medium green (unripe) tomatoes
⅓ cup stone-ground cornmeal
⅓ cup low-cho bake mix
½ teaspoon salt
¼ teaspoon pepper
3 tablespoons vegetable oil or ghee (ghee is better, for flavor and crispness)
tartar sauce or remoulade

1. Slice the tomatoes ½ inch thick. On a plate, combine the cornmeal, bake mix, salt, and pepper. Press the tomato slices into the mixture to coat.
2. Heat the oil in a large nonstick skillet over medium-low heat. Fry the tomatoes for 8 to 10 minutes on a side, until golden. Drain on a wire rack or pat dry with paper towels. Serve with tartar sauce or remoulade.

SERVES 4.

CHUNKY CHILI CHICKEN

¼ cup olive oil
1½ pounds chicken thighs, skinned and boned, cut in ¾-inch chunks
1 red bell pepper, diced
1 small onion, chopped
3 cloves garlic, minced
1½ teaspoons cumin seeds
15 ounces chicken broth
15 ounces low-carbohydrate tomato sauce

1 can (10 ounces) whole tomatoes and green chilies, crushed
1 tablespoon chili powder
½ teaspoon dried oregano
⅛ teaspoon salt
⅛ teaspoon pepper
¼ cup sliced ripe olives
2 teaspoons cilantro
1 avocado, diced
½ cup grated cheddar cheese

1. In a Dutch oven or large, heavy saucepan, heat 3 tablespoons of the oil over medium-high heat. Sauté the chicken until browned, about 8 minutes.
2. Remove the chicken to a bowl, wipe out the pan, and heat the remaining oil. Sauté the bell pepper, onion, garlic, and cumin about 5 minutes, until the onion is soft. Add the chicken broth, tomato sauce, tomatoes and chilies, oregano, salt, and pepper and mix well. Stir in the chicken and any juices. Cover, reduce the heat, and simmer for 20 minutes.
3. Stir the olives into the chili and simmer for 15 minutes. Add the cilantro. Serve in bowls and sprinkle with the avocado and cheese.

SERVES 6.

BLUEBERRY SCONES

2 cups low-carbohydrate bake mix
2 teaspoons baking powder
1 tablespoon fresh lemon zest
½ teaspoon salt

2 packets sugar substitute
2 cups fresh blueberries
1 cup sour cream
2 eggs
3 tablespoons butter, melted and cooled

1. Heat the oven to 350°. In a mixing bowl, whisk together the bake mix, baking powder, lemon zest, salt, and sugar substitute. Add blueberries and mix gently.
2. In a separate bowl, whisk together the sour cream, eggs, and butter. Combine the wet and dry ingredients.
3. On an ungreased cookie sheet, pat the dough into an 8-inch circle. Cut it into 8 wedges. Bake for 55 minutes, covering with foil after 25 minutes if necessary, until golden brown.

MAKES 8 SCONES.

JAMAICAN JERKED BEEF

4 small jalapeño or serrano chilies
2 teaspoons allspice
½ teaspoon cinnamon
⅛ teaspoon freshly grated nutmeg
1½ teaspoons paprika
1 teaspoon salt
½ teaspoon pepper
4 scallions, white part and 2 inches of green, cut into ½-inch pieces
2 tablespoons cider vinegar
1 tablespoon vegetable oil
4 boneless chuck eye beauty steaks (about 8 ounces each), ¾ inch thick

1. Wearing rubber gloves, remove the tips from the chilies. Cut them in half lengthwise; remove and save the seeds and veins. Cut the chilies into small pieces.

2. In a food processor, combine the chilies, allspice, cinnamon, nutmeg, paprika, salt, pepper, and scallions. Process for 20 seconds. Scrape the sides of the bowl with a rubber spatula. Add the vinegar and oil. Process the mixture until it forms a paste, about 20 seconds. Taste the mixture. Add ½ teaspoon (or more) of the reserved chili seeds and veins, if desired, to increase heat level.

3. Brush the steaks on both sides with 1½ tablespoons of the "jerk" mixture. Cover with plastic wrap and refrigerate for 2 to 4 hours.

4. A half hour before cooking, remove the steaks from the refrigerator and prepare the grill or heat the broiler. Grill the steaks until seared and well crusted on one side, about 5 minutes. Turn and cook 4 to 5 minutes more for medium rare to medium.

5. Thin the remaining "jerk" paste with a little water until it is the consistency of a sauce, heat, and serve with the steaks.

SERVES 4.

CORNED BEEF HASH

3 cups leftover corned beef, cubed
2 cups cooked, cubed turnips
½ cup chopped onion
½ cup heavy cream
3 tablespoons vegetable oil or butter

1. Mix the beef and turnips in a bowl. Add the onion and heavy cream and stir.

2. Heat the oil in a heavy nonstick skillet over medium-low heat for 1 minute. Add the hash mixture and cook until a bottom crust forms, about 10 minutes. Turn over and brown the other side. Serve with fried eggs, if desired.

SERVES 4.

CHICKEN CACCIATORE

3 tablespoons extra-virgin olive oil
1 fryer chicken (3 to 3½ pounds), cut into 8 pieces
1 small onion, thinly sliced
2 garlic cloves, minced
2 teaspoons dried rosemary
½ cup dry white wine
¾ teaspoon salt
¼ teaspoon crushed red pepper flakes
1½ cups canned plum tomatoes, drained and coarsely chopped

1. In a large skillet, heat the oil over medium-high heat. Cook the chicken in two batches, skin side down, until browned, about 8 minutes. Remove the chicken to a plate. Add the onion, garlic, and rosemary to the skillet and cook until the onion is softened, about 4 minutes. Add the wine and heat until boiling, stirring to loosen any browned bits from the bottom. Add the salt and pepper flakes.
2. Return the chicken to the pan, skin side up, adding any juices from the plate. Boil until almost all the wine has evaporated, about 2 minutes, turning the chicken once. Add the tomatoes and turn the chicken over to skin side up. Cover, reduce the heat to low, and simmer until

the chicken is cooked through, about 30 minutes.

3. Remove the chicken to a serving platter. Heat the cooking liquid to boiling over high heat. Boil about 2 minutes to thicken. Spoon the sauce over the chicken.

SERVES 4.

PINEAPPLE-RICOTTA PANCAKES

3 large eggs
3 tablespoons low-carbohydrate bake mix
salt
⅓ cup heavy cream
¾ cup ricotta cheese
¼ cup fresh pineapple, diced
1 packet sugar substitute such as Splenda
1½ tablespoons butter

1. In a bowl, whisk the eggs, bake mix, and salt until smooth. Gradually whisk in the cream. Let stand for 5 minutes.

2. Press the ricotta through a fine sieve and add the pineapple and sugar substitute. Reserve.

3. Melt the butter in a small nonstick skillet over medium heat. Pour in 2 tablespoons of the batter and tilt the pan or spread the batter to coat the bottom. Cook until golden on the bottom, then turn over and cook 1 minute more. Remove the pancake to a plate, and repeat with the remaining batter.

4. Spread the pancakes with the ricotta-pineapple mixture and roll up.

SERVES 4.

BAKED RATATOUILLE

⅓ cup olive oil
4 garlic cloves, minced
1 teaspoon salt
½ teaspoon dried rosemary
½ teaspoon dried thyme
¼ teaspoon pepper
1 small eggplant (about 1¼ pounds), cut into 1-inch cubes
1 medium zucchini, cut into 1-inch cubes
1 yellow squash, cut into 1-inch cubes
1 small red pepper, cut into ½-inch pieces
1 small tomato, cut into ½-inch cubes
1 small onion, thinly sliced

1. Heat the oven to 425°. Place all the ingredients in a 10-inch by 15-inch baking dish. Toss until the vegetables are coated evenly with the oil.
2. Cover the dish with foil and bake for 15 minutes. Uncover and cook for 30 minutes more, stirring occasionally, until the vegetables are tender and browned.

SERVES 6.

CAJUN CHICKEN WITH OKRA

4 teaspoons vegetable oil
2 pounds chicken thighs, skinned and boned, cut into 1½-inch pieces
29 ounces (2 cans) Cajun-style stewed tomatoes, undrained, chopped

4 cloves garlic, minced
1⅓ cups low-sodium chicken broth
½ teaspoon salt
½ teaspoon crushed red pepper flakes
20 ounces frozen cut okra, thawed
4 tablespoons water
3 tablespoons low-carbohydrate bake mix
½ teaspoon hot red pepper sauce

1. In a large nonstick skillet, heat the oil over medium-high heat until hot. Add the chicken. Cook until browned on all sides, about 5 minutes. Add the tomatoes, garlic, chicken broth, salt, and pepper flakes and heat until boiling. Cover, reduce the heat, and simmer until the chicken is cooked through, about 12 minutes. Add the okra. Cover and simmer about 3 minutes.
2. Combine the water and the bake mix in a small bowl and mix until blended. Whisk into the chicken mixture and simmer, uncovered, until thick, about 2 minutes. Add the hot pepper sauce.

SERVES 4.

ASPARAGUS AND LEEK SOUP

2 tablespoons butter
1 leek (white part only), halved lengthwise, washed, and chopped
¾ pound asparagus, cut into ½-inch pieces
2 cups chicken stock
⅓ cup heavy cream
salt
pepper

1. Heat the butter in a large saucepan over medium-high heat until the foam subsides. Add the leek and sauté, stirring, for 2 minutes. Add the asparagus and sauté, stirring, for 1 minute.
2. Add the chicken stock and bring to a boil. Lower the heat, cover, and simmer until the asparagus is tender, about 8 to 10 minutes.
3. Place the soup in a food processor. Add the cream, salt, and pepper and puree for 1 minute, or until smooth. Serve immediately.

SERVES 4.

THAI BEEF GRILL

4 beef top loin steaks or 2 boneless top sirloin steaks, 1 inch thick, well trimmed
6 tablespoons light low-carbohydrate teriyaki sauce
2 small onions, cut into ½-inch slices

Peanut Sauce:
4 tablespoons creamy no-sugar peanut butter
¼ to ½ teaspoon red pepper flakes
4 tablespoons low-carbohydrate teriyaki sauce
4 tablespoons water

1. Prepare the grill or broiler. Brush both sides of the steaks with 6 tablespoons of teriyaki sauce. Grill the steaks and the onion over medium-hot coals, turning occasionally, for 15 to 18 minutes (a little longer for top loin steak) for medium-rare to medium.
2. While the steak is cooking, make the peanut sauce. Combine the peanut butter and red pepper flakes in a small bowl. Using a fork, gradually stir in 4 tablespoons

of teriyaki sauce and the water, mixing until smooth.
3. Slice the steaks crosswise into thick slices. Serve with
the onion slices and peanut sauce.

SERVES 4.

22

YOUR AGE-DEFYING VITANUTRIENT PLAN

It is a happy fact that the arena of vitanutrient supplements sees breakthroughs and new developments practically every day. The mere fact that serious studies of vitanutrients are now commonplace is very encouraging to me and my many colleagues in complementary medicine. It is increasingly difficult for the medical establishment to persist in ignoring the incontrovertible results of these studies, especially when statistics show that adverse drug reactions directly cause more than 100,000 deaths a year and are implicated in many more.

The point, however, is not the adverse effects of drugs so much as the importance of various vitanutrients for maintaining and improving your health. And here the picture is very promising indeed, as all the breakthroughs and developments confirm.

The goal of your age-defying program, of course, is to help you achieve your maximum life expectancy with minimum disability. A vitanutrient plan will help. But just as no one diet fits all, vitanutrient needs also vary from person to person; moreover, these needs change somewhat throughout your lifetime. So in this chapter, I'll offer first a basic nutrition vitamin and mineral formula that's appropriate for almost all adults, then suggestions for vitanutrients that can address specific health issues. This should provide the basis of a flexible supplement program appropriate for most people.

Be aware also that there's no need to purchase each individual supplement and take each one separately. Many reputable manufacturers now make well-designed formulas that include many or most of the basic vitanutrients in dosages large enough to be effective. Among them is the prototypical formula I developed for my Atkins Center patients, which is available to readers at many health food stores. In addition, many reputable manufacturers make formulas for treating specific health issues, such as osteoporosis or high blood pressure, just as I do at the Atkins Center. Your best bet, therefore, is to select a supplement that gives you the maximum breadth and dosage possible, then add whatever other individual vitanutrients that are appropriate for your own physical and medical profile.*

BASIC VITANUTRIENTS

The formula in Table 22.1 is designed as a basic nutrition vitamin/mineral formula for adults. A few words of explanation are in order.

First, when selecting a combined vitamin/mineral supplement, bear in mind that outdated and pointless FDA regulations limit the amount of folic acid in any supplement to 800 mcg. To get the full 3 to 4 grams of folic acid that are necessary for optimal health, you will need to take additional over-the-counter folic acid supplements, or ask your doctor to prescribe a larger amount.

In addition, in order to make basic formulas less

---

*While I don't have the space here to give detailed discussions of the vitanutrients listed, many have been discussed in earlier chapters of this book. For detailed information, however, please see *Dr. Atkins' Vita-Nutrient Solution*.

Table 22.1

BASIC NUTRITION VITAMIN/MINERAL FORMULA	
VITANUTRIENT	DAILY INTAKE
Natural beta-carotene	3,000–6,000 IU
Vitamin A	1,500–3,000 IU
Vitamin B_1	30–60 mg
Vitamin B_2	24–48 mg
Niacin	15–30 mg
Niacinamide	30–60 mg
Pantothenic acid	75–150 mg
Pantethine	75–150 mg
Vitamin B_6	30–60 mg
Folic acid	2,000–4,000 mcg
Biotin	225–450 mcg
Vitamin B_{12}	180–240 mcg
Vitamin C	500–1,000 mg
Vitamin D_2	90–180 IU
Vitamin E	150–300 IU
Copper	600–1,200 mcg
Magnesium	50–100 mg
Calcium	200–400 mg
Choline	300–600 mg
Inositol	240–480 mg
PABA	300–600 mg
Manganese	12–24 mg
Zinc	24–48 mg
Citrus bioflavonoids	450–600 mg
Chromium	150–300 mcg
Selenium	120–240 mcg
N-acetyl-cysteine	60–120 mg
Molybdenum	30–60 mcg
Vanadyl sulfate	45–90 mcg
Octacosanol	450–900 mcg
Reduced glutathione	15–30 mg

bulky, many manufacturers provide less than the minimum requirement for calcium. If you select such a formula and your dietary calcium intake is low, you should include a 500-mg calcium tablet as part of your basic program. For best results, choose supplements made with calcium citrate or calcium lactate.

Also, when you select vitamin E supplements, choose only the natural kind.

Finally, in addition to your daily dose of vitamins and minerals, I recommend daily supplements of the essential fatty acids discussed in detail in Chapter 14. The optimal dose is 400 mg each of borage oil (GLA), fish oil (EPA and DHA), and flaxseed oil (ALA), taken two to three times daily for a total of 800 to 1,200 mg of each. Many manufacturers make a combined essential oils formula that contains all three forms.

With that as a preface, have a look at the basic nutrition formula of Table 22.1. It's designed to help you maintain basic good health *and* prevent many of the preventable diseases of aging.

VITANUTRIENT SOLUTIONS

In addition to the basic formula, you'll want to take vitanutrient supplements that address your own specific health issues. The protocols that follow let you do just that, with a particular supplement and/or formula plus dosage suggested to prevent and/or treat each of ten major health concerns.

To augment any of these supplements to reach the higher doses suggested in the protocols, subtract the amount of the vitanutrient in your daily formula from the larger amount in the protocol. The difference is the amount of the vitanutrient you need to add.

HEART AND VASCULAR HEALTH

Antioxidants, both from diet and from supplements, are extremely important for preventing heart disease and protecting your coronary arteries. You also need to maintain high levels of folic acid to remove artery-damaging homocysteine from your system efficiently.

To make your homocysteine level perfect, the first step is diagnosis. A homocysteine blood test is easily obtained, and diagnosis is linear, meaning that the higher the level of homocysteine in the blood, even in the "normal" range, the more urgent is the need to provide the necessary vitamins. Most people with readings of 8 μmol/L should take the supplements, and anyone whose reading is over 12 μmol/L absolutely *must* take them.

The three vitamins that can lower your homocysteine level are all B vitamins. All three are quite safe to take in the dosages I recommend to my patients: 100 mg of B_6, 2,000 mcg of B_{12}, and 10 mg of folic acid. A recent study showed that a program with only 5 mg of folic acid and only 500 mcg of B_{12} failed to reduce homocysteine levels nearly one-third of the time.[1] (See Chapter 4 for more on heart health and homocysteine.)

In addition to perfecting your homocysteine level, the vitanutrients in Table 22.2 are valuable for maximizing your overall heart health, as has been discussed throughout this book. Use them to augment the basic vitanutrient formula.

Table 22.2

| VITANUTRIENTS FOR HEART AND VASCULAR HEALTH ||
VITANUTRIENT	DAILY INTAKE
Magnesium	400–800 mg
Coenzyme Q_{10}	60–120 mg
L-carnitine	1,000–2,000 mg
Taurine	500–1,000 mg
Vitamin E	400–800 IU
Vitamin C	1,000–3,000 mg
Essential oils formula	3,600–7,200 mg
Mixed tocotrienols	100–200 mg
Chromium	200–400 mcg
Natural beta-carotene	25,000 IU
Ginkgo biloba	240–480 mg
B complex	25–50 mg
Folic acid	3–6 mg

HIGH CHOLESTEROL

As has been discussed in detail throughout this book, your total cholesterol level alone is not a particularly accurate indicator of your risk of heart disease or stroke. A much better marker is your ratio of HDL cholesterol to triglycerides. In my experience, there is rarely if ever a need for lipid-lowering drugs to reduce your LDL cholesterol, raise your HDL cholesterol, and improve your ratio of HDL to triglycerides. The vitanutrients in Table 22.3, in combination with a low-carbohydrate diet, should easily lower your total cholesterol. To be sure the program is helping you, you must work with your physician to monitor your blood lipid levels on a regular basis.

To help improve your ratio of triglycerides to HDL cholesterol, follow the high-cholesterol formula and add: carnitine, 1,500–3,000 mg daily; EPA/DHA from fish

Table 22.3

VITANUTRIENTS FOR HIGH TOTAL CHOLESTEROL	
VITANUTRIENT	DAILY INTAKE
Pantethine	600–1,200 mg
Inositol hexanicotinate	500–1,500 mg
Chromium	300–600 mcg
Essential oils formula	7,200 mg
Vitamin C	1,000–5,000 mg
Mixed fiber supplement	10 g
Lecithin granules	2–3 tbsp
Guggulipid	100–200 mg
Borage oil (GLA)	1,200–3,600 mg
Garlic	2,400–4,000 mg
Gamma oryzanol	300–600 mg
Mixed tocotrienols	200–400 mg
Natural beta-carotene	25,000–50,000 IU

oil, 1,200–2,400 mg daily; chromium, 400–800 mcg daily; and vanadyl sulfate, 15–30 mg daily.

HIGH BLOOD PRESSURE

To this day, researchers still aren't precisely sure why some people have hypertension, or high blood pressure. But it is a fact that your blood pressure tends to rise as you get older, a tendency that must be counteracted as part of your age-defying program. The best way to do that is through the low-carbohydrate diet in combination with the vitanutrients listed in Table 22.4.

BLOOD SUGAR IMBALANCES

As you must surely appreciate by now, it's my view that blood sugar imbalances are the most important

Table 22.4

VITANUTRIENTS FOR HYPERTENSION	
VITANUTRIENT	DAILY INTAKE
Taurine	1,500–3,000 mg
Magnesium	500–1,000 mg
Hawthorn	240–480 mg
Potassium aspartate	400–800 mg
Vitamin B_6	100–200 mg
Essential oils formula	3,600–7,200 mg
Garlic	2,400–3,200 mg
Coenzyme Q_{10}	100–200 mg
Carnitine	500–1,000 mg
Chromium	300–600 mcg

nutrition-based diseases in the Western world—and they are becoming the most important in many parts of the developing world as well. The incidence of diabetes is exploding worldwide, with billions of new cases expected over the next few decades. And while diabetes is a major disease in its own right, it is also a major risk factor for coronary heart disease, stroke, kidney disease, and other serious complications. (For a thorough discussion of the entire issue of blood sugar, insulin, and the stages leading up to diabetes, refer back to Chapter 5.)

Here I give two protocols for preventing the blood sugar imbalances that can lead to prediabetes and/or the disease itself. Table 22.5 lists vitanutrients that help keep the blood sugar in balance and ameliorate or prevent early prediabetes and early type II diabetes. Table 22.6 is for prediabetics who need to bring elevated blood sugar down to normal levels and for type II diabetics who are now taking antidiabetes medications.

Table 22.5

VITANUTRIENTS FOR PREDIABETICS	
VITANUTRIENT	DAILY INTAKE
Chromium	200–600 mcg
Zinc	50–100 mg
Magnesium	300–600 mg
Lipoic acid	150–300 mg
Coenzyme Q_{10}	45–90 mg
Biotin	2–4 mg
Essential oils formula	7,200 mg
Selenium	100–200 mcg
Vitamin B_6	75–150 mg

OVERWEIGHT AND OBESITY

More than half of all adult Americans are overweight; more than a quarter of all American children are overweight. In the long run, these figures will translate into widespread, extremely expensive poor health, lost productivity and pleasure in life, and early death.

Table 22.6

VITANUTRIENTS FOR DIABETICS	
VITANUTRIENT	DAILY INTAKE
Chromium	500–1,000 mcg
Vanadyl sulfate	30–60 mg
Coenzyme Q_{10}	90–180 mg
Biotin	7.5–15 mg
Inositol	800–1,600 mg
Zinc	90–180 mg
Niacinamide	30–600 mg
DHEA	20–40 mg

Severe weight gain is actually a manifestation of insulin resistance, as discussed at length in Chapter 5. To counteract the tendency, your best bet is the low-carbohydrate, high-protein diet strategy that has worked for thousands of my patients and for the millions of people who have followed the advice in *Dr. Atkins' New Diet Revolution*. The diet alone *will* cause you to lose weight. Combine it with the vitanutrients in Table 22.7, however, and you can open up blocked metabolic pathways and facilitate your weight loss.

BRAIN NUTRIENTS

Keeping your cognitive abilities high is so important a part of your age-defying program that I devoted all of Chapter 18 to a discussion of vitanutrients that help. Table 22.8 gives you the basic protocol for getting started on boosting your brain power.

Table 22.7

VITANUTRIENTS FOR WEIGHT LOSS	
VITANUTRIENT	DAILY INTAKE
Chromium	400–800 mcg
Carnitine	1,000–2,000 mg
Coenzyme Q_{10}	75–150 mg
Glutamine	2–4 g
Phenylalanine	750–1,500 mg
Choline	750–1,500 mg
Inositol	1,000–2,000 mg
Methionine	400–800 mg
Lipoic acid	100–300 mg

Table 22.8

BRAIN VITANUTRIENTS	
VITANUTRIENT	DAILY INTAKE
Thiamin	50–100 mg
Folic acid	3–6 mg
Phosphatidyl serine	200–400 mg
Phosphatidyl choline	200–400 mg
Ginkgo biloba (standardized extract)	120–240 mg
Acetyl-l-carnitine	100–200 mg
Octacosanol	10–20 mg
Vitamin B_{12}	1,000–2,000 mcg
Vitamin B_6	30–60 mg

MENOPAUSE SYMPTOMS

Contrary to the gospel as espoused by the medical establishment, the discomforts of menopause do not need to be treated with hormone replacement therapy. As I discussed in Chapter 13, there are safer alternatives to HRT, and these alternatives have no side effects. In fact, vitanutrients like those in the protocol in Table 22.9 are extremely helpful at this time in a woman's life, when she needs optimal nutrition.

Once again, I must repeat that the large doses of folic acid recommended in Table 22.9 are best obtained with a doctor's prescription. But women who need to shrink uterine fibroids, prevent breast cancer recurrences, or deal with endometriosis or fibrocystic breasts should keep their dose of supplemental folic acid below 600 mcg daily.

Also, the recommendations for pregnenolone and DHEA are based on the dosages most women need, but you should work with your physician to identify your current blood levels and determine the amounts that will restore your levels to those of a thirty-year-old.

Table 22.9

VITANUTRIENTS FOR MENOPAUSE SYMPTOMS	
VITANUTRIENT	DAILY INTAKE
Folic acid	20–60 mg
Boron	6–18 mg
Pregnenolone	30–60 mg
DHEA	20–40 mg
Essential oils formula	3,600–7,200 mg
Vitamin E	400–1,200 iu
Vitamin B_6	150–300 mg
Gamma oryzanol	150–450 mg
B vitamin complex	50–100 mg
Chromium	200–600 mcg

PREVENTING AND TREATING OSTEOPOROSIS

Osteoporosis—thin, brittle bones that break easily—is a disease that is easily slowed or even prevented. A combination of exercise, natural hormones, and vitanutrients can be very helpful for dealing with this crippling disease. In general, the vitanutrients in Table 22.10, when combined with exercise, will help prevent and treat osteoporosis just as well as the powerful drugs that are commonly prescribed. When choosing a calcium supplement, select one made with calcium citrate or calcium lactate for maximum absorption. As for the doses of folic acid and the hormones DHEA and pregnenolone, the same recommendations hold true here as for menopause symptoms.

Table 22.10

VITANUTRIENTS FOR OSTEOPOROSIS	
VITANUTRIENT	DAILY INTAKE
Folic acid	20–60 mg
Boron	6–12 mg
Calcium	800–1,600 mg
Vitamin D	400–800 IU
Magnesium	400–800 mg
Vitamin K	150–300 mcg
Silicon	100–300 mg
Lysine	500–1,000 mg
B vitamin complex	500–1,000 mg
Ipriflavone	300–600 mg

PROSTATE PROTECTION

By the time a typical man reaches the age of sixty or so, he is quite likely to be experiencing the symptoms of benign enlargement of the prostate, also known as benign prostate hypertrophy, or BPH. This condition, in which the prostate gland becomes swollen enough to obstruct urine flow, makes urination difficult and causes frequent trips to the bathroom during the night. When frequent awakenings interfere with restful sleep, this may actually cause a decline in your production in growth hormone, to say nothing of the tiredness the next day.

Standard medical treatment for BPH begins with strong drugs that often have unwanted side effects. The treatment typically then proceeds to complication-laden, often unnecessary surgery that can leave the patient incontinent and impotent. The vitanutrient approach in Table 22.11 is far less harsh, which is also excellent for supporting male reproductive health in general. Plan on taking the supplements for at least three months before you notice a major improvement in your symptoms.

Table 22.11

VITANUTRIENTS FOR MALE REPRODUCTIVE HEALTH	
VITANUTRIENT	DAILY INTAKE
Saw palmetto (standardized extract)	250–500 mg
Pygeum africanum (standardized extract)	100–200 mg
Glutamic acid	50–100 mg
Glycine	250–500 mg
Alanine	250–500 mg
Manganese	20–40 mg
Essential oils formula	3,600–7,200 mg
Zinc	50–100 mg

With the tables in this and the previous chapter, you have the tools you need to arm yourself for the fight against aging. In the final chapter, we'll put it all together—then we'll go forth and do battle.

23

The age-defying steps I've outlined in this book are designed to help you live a longer, healthier life. They're based on my years of clinical experience, combined with the latest cutting-edge research. There's nothing mysterious or difficult about my age-defying approach. The basic diet is easy to understand and even easier to follow. The vitanutrients I recommend and the other age-defying techniques I suggest are based on proven medicine and can be used by anyone. There's every reason to think that you too can benefit from them.

The world of age-defying research is very dynamic and exciting. In fact, it is so dynamic that your conventional physician may not be aware of the latest developments and may not understand all the age-defying techniques I've discussed. Any conscientious, knowledgeable, and open-minded physician should be able to work with you to achieve at least some of your age-defying goals. Here are some thoughts on how to go about it.

WORKING WITH YOUR DOCTOR

If, as I talked about how to use laboratory tests to determine your blood lipids, insulin level, hormone levels, and more, you thought to yourself, "I'm going to need a doctor to get the tests done," you were absolutely right. Only a physician can do the sort of testing you need and interpret the results for you, and only a physician can supervise some of the techniques I suggest.

To get the most from the age-defying concepts I've discussed, you not only need to know about the workings of your own body, you also need to work with your doctor to verify that the changes you make in your diet, vitanutrient use, and lifestyle are having the desired effect.

It would be ideal if you could find a doctor who is conversant with—and practices—the information in this book. Such doctors are rare, but many of them belong to such organizations as the Foundation for the Advancement of Innovative Medicine (FAIM) at (877) 634-3246 or www.faim.org and the American College for Advancement in Medicine (ACAM) at (800) 532-3688 or www.acam.org. You can contact these organizations to provide you with a list of their membership.

If you encounter an open-minded physician who practices complementary medicine and helps you achieve better health, please contact me so that I can put the doctor's name on our referral list.

CHANGING THE WORLD OF HEALTH

I dedicated this book to my followers for a reason. I believe that what is really needed to transform today's medicine is a group of people who consider themselves my supporters, followers, adherents, or, as some people have called themselves, Atkids. Lest you think this is self-serving, please bear in mind that I have dedicated my life to making the world better for the people whose paths cross mine. What we need are people who can help change the medical establishment—a grassroots movement that ensures that the truth about health, instead of mainstream propaganda, gets out to everyone.

The most convincing argument we can deliver is our success in achieving the goal of this book: having a longer, healthier life span.

If you'd like to help effect the necessary changes in our society, I ask you to let us know who you are. Visit our interactive Web site at www.atkinscenter.com or call The Atkins Center at 888 ATKINS 8. We want to know how you are doing as you follow the age-defying lifestyle. Send us your case histories, your experiences, and your comments.

ONE LAST WORD

Today the breakthroughs in age-defying medicine come so frequently that I was adding information to this book until the absolute last possible moment. The cutting-edge research I discuss is the most up-to-date I could find. Yet in the short time it took to print this volume and get it into your hands, there doubtless will have been new scientific developments that could change your life for the better. As new developments arise in this fascinating area, I will be telling you about them on my Web site and in my newsletter, *Dr. Atkins' Health Revelations*.

Communication has been revolutionized by the Internet, so no longer does an author such as myself simply write a book and hope that people will read it and take its message to heart. Today the author and his readers can have a true interactive relationship. I welcome your comments and questions and look forward, with the help of my staff, to answering them. I hope you will be one of those people whose age-defying success serves as a role model for many more. That way, the movement toward making us all healthier, all more long-lived, will prevail.

APPENDIX

GLYCEMIC INDEX OF COMMON FOODS

The glycemic index (GI) measures the effect a particular food has on your blood sugar when you eat it. Foods that are high on the glycemic index raise your blood sugar higher than foods that are lower on the index. The standard against which foods are measured for the glycemic index is glucose, otherwise known as table sugar, which is given the rating GI 100. The glycemic index concept applies only to high-carbohydrate foods—foods that are high in protein or fat don't raise your blood sugar much, if at all. The glycemic index is a useful tool for selecting foods for your age-defying diet—just look for foods that are as low on the index as possible. Bear in mind, however, that the index doesn't take into account factors that slow down how quickly a food raises your blood sugar. If you have some grapes (GI 45) for dessert after eating a high-protein meal, the fructose from the grapes will enter your system more slowly and thus raise your blood sugar more slowly as well.

The Glycemic Index of Common Foods

FOOD	RATING	FOOD	RATING
Maltose	110	Spaghetti	50
Glucose	100	Oatmeal	49
Baked potato	98	Grapes	45
Carrots	92	Orange	40
Honey	87	Apple	39
Cornflakes	80	Tomato	38
Whole-wheat bread	72	Chickpeas	36
White rice	72	Lima beans	36
White bread	69	Yogurt	36
Shredded wheat	67	Whole milk	34
Brown rice	66	Pears	34
Raisins	64	Skim milk	32
Beets	64	Kidney beans	29
Bananas	62	Lentils	29
Corn	59	Grapefruit	26
Green peas	51	Plum	25
Potato chips	51	Cherries	23
Sweet potato	51	Peanuts	13

NOTES

Chapter 2

1. Morbidity and Mortality Weekly Report 1999; 48:664–68.
2. Cohen A M, Fidel J, Cohen B et al. Diabetes, blood lipids, lipoproteins, and change of environment: restudy of the "new immigrant Yemenites" in Israel. Metabolism 1979; 28:716–28.
3. Al-Nuaim A R. Prevalence of glucose intolerance in urban and rural communities in Saudi Arabia. Diabet Med 1997; 14:595–602.
4. World Health Organization statistics; King, H, Aubert R E, Herman W H. Global burden of diabetes, 1995–2025: prevalence, numerical estimates, and projections. Diabetes Care 1998; 21:1414–31.

Chapter 3

1. U.S. Bureau of Census.
2. Castelli W P. Concerning the possibility of a nutritional . . . Arch Intern Med 1992; 152:1371–72.
3. Morbidity and Mortality Weekly Report 1999; 48:664–68.
4. Resource Utilization Among Congestive Heart Failure (REACH) Study statistics, March 1999; American Heart Association statistics September 1999.
5. Statistics from American Heart Association, based on National Heart, Lung, and Blood Institute studies.
6. De Backer G et al. Lifetime-risk prediction: a complicated business. Lancet 1999; 353:82–83, 89–92.

Chapter 4

1. Stampfer M J, Krauss R M, Ma J et al. A prospective study of triglyceride level, low-density lipoprotein particle diameter, and risk of myocardial infarction. JAMA 1996; 276:882–88.

2. Bass K M, Newschaffer C J, Klag M J, Bush T L. Plasma lipoprotein levels as predictors of cardiovascular death in women. Arch Intern Med 1993; 153:2209–16.

3. Presentation by K Moysich, annual meeting International Society for Environmental Epidemiology, 7 September 1999.

4. Stampfer M J, Krauss R M, Ma J et al. A prospective study of triglyceride level, low-density lipoprotein particle diameter, and risk of myocardial infarction. JAMA 1996; 276:882–88.

5. Assmann G, Schulte H. The importance of triglycerides: results from the Prospective Cardiovascular Muenster (PROCAM) Study. Eur J Epidemiol 1992; Supplement 1:99–103; Assmann G, Schulte H. Relation of high-density lipoprotein cholesterol and triglycerides to incidence of atherosclerotic coronary artery disease (the PROCAM experience). Am J Cardiology 1992; 70:733–37.

6. Gaziano J M et al. Fasting triglycerides, high-density lipoprotein, and risk of myocardial infarction. Circulation 1997; 96: 2520–25.

7. Reissell P K et al. Treatment of hypertriglyceridemia. Am J Clin Nutr 1966; 19:84–98.

8. Sanchez-Delgado E, Liechti H. Lifetime risk of developing coronary heart disease. Lancet 1999; 353:934.

9. Rath M, Pauling L. Immunological evidence for the accumulation of lipoprotein(a) in the atherosclerotic lesion of the hypoascorbemic guinea pig. Proc Natl Acad Sci USA 1990; 87:9388–90.

10. Fenech M. Towards promulgation of the healthy life span. Ann NY Acad Sci 1997; 854:23–36.

11. Graham I M, Daly L E, Refsum H M et al. Plasma homocysteine as a risk factor for vascular disease. The European Concerted Action Project. JAMA 1997; 277:1775–81.

12. Kark J D, Selhub J, Adler B et al. Nonfasting plasma total homocysteine level and mortality in middle-aged and elderly men and women in Jerusalem. Ann Intern Med 1999; 131: 321–30.

13. American Heart Association recommendation, Homocysteine, Folic Acid and Cardiovascular Disease, 1998.

Chapter 5

1. Perls T T, Silver M H. Living to 100. NY: Basic Books, 1998, 113.

2. Cerami A, Vlassare H, Brownlee M. Glucose and aging. Scientific American 1987; 256:90–96.

3. Diabetes Care 1999; 22:45–49.

4. Tominaga M, Fguchi H, Manaka H et al. Impaired glucose tolerance is a risk factor for cardiovascular disease, but not impaired fasting glucose: the Funagata diabetes study. Diabetes Care 1999; 22:920–24.

5. Smith M A et al. Advanced Maillard reaction end products are associated with Alzheimer disease pathology. Proc Nat Acad Sci USA 1994; 91:5710–14 and Vitek M P et al. Advance glycation end products contribute to amyloidosis in Alzheimer disease. Proc Nat Acad Sci USA 1994; 91:4766–70.

6. Bucala R et al. Modification of low density lipoprotein by advanced glycation end products contributes to the dyslipidemia of diabetes and renal insufficiency. Proc Nat Acad Sci USA 1994; 91:9441–45.

7. Al-Abed Y et al. Inhibition of advanced glycation endproduct formation by acetaldehyde: role in the cardioprotective effect of ethanol. Proc Nat Acad Sci USA 1999; 96:2385–90.

8. Fournier A M, Gadia M T, Kubrusly D B et al. Blood pressure, insulin and glycemia in nondiabetic subjects. Am J Med 1983; 80:861–64.

9. Nestler J E, Beer N A, Jakubowicz J, Beer R M. Effects of a reduction in circulating insulin by metformin on serum dehydroepiandrosterone sulfate in nondiabetic men. J Clin Endocrinol Metab 1994; 78:549–54.

10. Buffington C K, Pourmotabbed G, Kitabchi A E. Case report: amelioration of insulin resistance in diabetes with dehydroepiandrosterone. Am J Med Sci 1993; 306:320–24.

11. Evans G W, Swensen G, Walters K. Chromium picolinate decreases calcium excretion and increases dehydroepiandrosterone (DHEA) in post menopausal women. FASEB J 1995; 9: A449.

Chapter 6

1. Harman, D. Free radical theory of aging: role of free radicals in the origination and evolution of life, aging, and disease processes. In John J E Jr, Walford R, Harman D et al., eds. Free Radicals, Aging and Degenerative Diseases. NY: Alan R. Liss, 1986, 3–49.

2. Harman, D. The biological clock: The mitochondria? J Am Geriatrics Soc 1972; 20:145–147.

3. Diplock A T. Antioxidant nutrients and disease prevention. Am J Clin Nutr 1991, 53:189S–193S.
4. Harman D. Aging: minimizing free radical damage. Journal of Anti-aging Medicine, 1999; 2:15–36.
5. Ibid.

Chapter 7

1. Weindruch, R, Walford R L, Figiel S, Guthrie D. The retardation of aging in mice by dietary restriction: longevity, cancer, immunity and lifetime energy intake. J Nutr 1986; 116: 641–54.
2. Walford R, Harris S B, Weindruch R. Dietary restriction and aging: historical phases, mechanisms, and current directions. J Nutr 1987; 117:1650–54.
3. Barzilai N, Gupta G. Revisiting the role of fat mass in the life extension induced by caloric restriction. J. Gerontol A Biol Sci Med Sci 1999; 54:B89–98.
4. Manson, J E et al. Body weight and mortality among women. NEJM 1995; 333:677–87.
5. Bloom W L, Azar G et al. Comparison of metabolic changes in fasting obese and lean patients. Ann NY Acad Sci 1965; 131:623–31.

Chapter 8

1. Hodis, H N, Mack W J, LaBree L et al. Serial coronary angiographic evidence that antioxidant vitamin intake reduces progression of coronary artery atherosclerosis. JAMA 1995; 273: 1849–54.
2. AHA statement January 1999.
3. Comstock G W, Burke A E, Hoffman S C et al. Serum concentrations of alpha tocopherol, beta carotene, and retinol preceding the diagnosis of rheumatoid arthritis and systemic lupus erythematosus. Ann Rheum Dis 1997; 56:323–25.
4. Rimm E B, Stampfer M J, Ascherio A et al. Vitamin E consumption and the risk of coronary heart disease in men. NEJM 1993; 328:1450–56.
5. Stampfer M J, Hennekens C H, Manson J E et al. Vitamin E consumption and the risk of coronary disease in women. NEJM 1993; 328:1444–49.
6. Stephens N G, Parsons A, Schofield P M et al. Randomised controlled study of vitamin E in patients with coronary disease:

Cambridge Heart Antioxidant Study (CHAOS). Lancet 1996; 347:781–86.

7. Azen S P, Qian D, Mack W J et al. Effect of supplementary antioxidant vitamin intake on carotid arterial wall intima-media thickness in a controlled clinical trial of cholesterol lowering. Circulation 1996; 94:2369–72.

8. Kushi L H, Folsom A R, Prineas R J et al. Dietary antioxidant vitamins and death from coronary heart disease in postmenopausal women. NEJM 1996; 334:1156–62.

9. Jialal I and Devaraj S. Arteriosclerosis, Thrombosis and Vascular Biology 1999; 19.

10. Nyssonone K, Parviainen M T, Salonen R et al. Vitamin C deficiency and risk of myocardial infarction: prospective population study of men from eastern Finland. BMJ 1997; 314: 634–38.

11. NHANES II.

12. Johnston C S, Thompson L L. Vitamin C status of an outpatient population. J Am Coll Nutr 1998; 17:366–70.

13. Vita J A et al. Low plasma ascorbic acid predicts the presence of an unstable coronary syndrome. J Am Coll Cardiology 1998; 31:980–86.

14. Podmore I D, Griffiths H R, Herbert K E et al. Vitamin C exhibits pro-oxidant properties. Nature 1998: 392:6676.

15. Duthie S J, Ma A, Ross M A, Collins A R. Antioxidant supplementation decreases oxidative DNA damage in human lymphocytes. Cancer Res 1996 56:1291–95.

16. Suadicani P, Hein H O, Gyntelberg F. Serum selenium concentration and risk of ischaemic heart disease in a prospective cohort study of 3000 males. Atherosclerosis 1992; 96:33–42.

17. Paleologos M, Cuming R G, Lazarus R. Cohort study of vitamin C intake and cognitive impairment. Am J Epidemiology 1998; 148:45–50.

18. Benson at annual meeting Amer Acad Neurology, 20 April 1999.

19. Schmidt R, Plasma antioxidants and cognitive performance in middle-aged and older adults: results of the Austrian Stroke Prevention Study. J Am Geriatrics Soc 1998; 46:1407–10.

20. Sano M, Ernesto C, Thomas R C, Klauber MR et al. A controlled trial of selegiline, alpha-tocopherol, or both as a treatment for Alzheimer's disease: the Alzheimer's disease cooperative study. NEJM 1997; 336:1216–22.

21. Ziegler D, Hanefeld M, Ruhnau K J et al. Treatment of symp-

tomatic diabetic peripheral neuropathy with the anti-oxidant alpha-lipoic acid. A 3-week multicenter randomized controlled trial (ALADIN Study). Diabetologica 1995; 38: 1425–33.

22. Henson D E, Block G, Levine M. Ascorbic acid: biologic functions and relation to cancer. J Natl Cancer Institute 1991; 83:547–50.

23. Block, G. Vitamin C and reduced mortality. Epidemiology 1992; 3:189–91.

24. Heinonen O P, Albanes D, Virtamo J et al. Prostate cancer and supplementation with alpha-tocopherol and beta-carotene: incidence and mortality in a controlled trial. J Natl Cancer Institute 1998; 90:440–46.

25. Clark L C et al. Effect of selenium supplementation for cancer prevention with carcinoma of the skin: a randomized controlled trial. JAMA 1996; 276:1957–63.

26. Colditz G A. Selenium and cancer prevention: promising results indicate further trials required. JAMA 1996; 276:1985.

27. Yoshizawa K, Willett W C, Morris S J et al. Study of prediagnostic selenium level in toenails and the risk of advanced prostate cancer. J Natl Cancer Institute 1998; 90:1219–24.

28. Leske M C, Chylack L T Jr, He Q et al. Antioxidant vitamins and nuclear opacity: the longitudinal study of cataract. Ophthalmology 1998; 105:831–36.

29. Seddon J M, Christen W G, Manson J E et al. The use of vitamin supplements and the risk of cataract among U.S. male physicians. Am J Pub Health 1994; 84:788–92.

30. Jacques P F, Taylor A, Hankinson S E et al. Long-term vitamin C supplement use and prevalence of early age-related lens opacities. Am J Clin Nutr 1997; 66:911–16.

31. Bendich A, Langseth L. The health effects of Vitamin C supplementation: a review. J Am Coll Nutr 1995; 14:124–136.

Chapter 9

1. Schnohr P, Thomsen O O, Riis Hansen P et al. Egg consumption and high-density-lipoprotein cholesterol. Journal of Internal Medicine 1994; 235:249–251.

2. Hu F B, Stampfer M, Rimm E B et al. A prospective study of egg consumption and risk of cardiovascular disease in men and women. JAMA 1999; 281:1387–94.

3. Beyer R E. The participation of coenzyme Q in free radical production and antioxidation. Free Radic Biol Med 1990; 8:

545–65; Lenaz G, Battino M, Castelluccio C et al. Studies on the role of ubiquinone in the control of the mitochondrial respiratory chain. Free Radical Research Communications 1990; 8:317–27.

4. Crane F L, Navas P. The diversity of coenzyme Q function. Mol Aspects Med 1997; 18:S1–6.

5. Esterbauer H, Striegl G, Puhl H, Rotheneder M. Continuous monitoring of in vitro oxidation of human low density lipoprotein. Free Radical Research Communications 1989; 6:67–75.

6. Reiter R J. Oxygen radical detoxification process during aging: the functional importance of melatonin. Aging (Milano) 1995; 5:340–51.

7. Poeggeler B, Reiter R J, Tan D X et al. Melatonin, hydroxyl radical-mediated oxidative damage, and aging: a hypothesis. J Pineal Res 1993; 14:151–68.

8. Reiter R J, Guerrero J M, Garcia J J, Acuña-Castroviejo D. Reactive oxygen intermediates, molecular damage, and aging. Relation to melatonin. Ann NY Acad Sci 1998; 854:410–24.

9. Brezinski A. Melatonin in humans. NEJM 1997; 336:186–95.

Chapter 10

1. Beecher G R, Khackik F. Qualitative relationship of dietary and plasma carotenoids in human beings. Ann NY Acad Sci 1992; 669:320–21.

2. Ford E S, Will J C, Bowman B A, Narayan K M. Diabetes mellitus and serum carotenoids: findings from the Third National Health and Nutrition Examination Survey. Am J Epidemiology 1999; 149:168–76.

3. Sies H, Stahl W. Vitamins E and C, beta-carotene, and other carotenoids as antioxidants. Am J Clin Nutr 1995; 62:1315S–21S.

4. Bendich A, Olson J A. Biological action of carotenoids. FASEB Journal 1989; 3:1927–32.

5. Gester H. Potential role of beta-carotene in the prevention of cardiovascular disease. International Journal of Vitamin and Nutrition Research 1991; 61:277–91.

6. Klipstein-Grobusch K, Geleijnse J M, den Breeijen J H et al. Dietary antioxidants and risk of myocardial infarction in the elderly: the Rotterdam Study. Am J Clin Nutr 1999; 69:261–66.

7. Diplock A T. Safety of antioxidant vitamins and beta-carotene. Am J Clin Nutr 1995; 62:1510S–16S.

8. Hennekens, C H, Buring J E, Manson J E et al. Lack of effect of long-term supplementation with beta-carotene on the incidence of malignant neoplasms and cardiovascular disease. NEJM 1996; 334:1145–90.

9. Omenn G S, Goodman G E, Thornquist M D et al. Effects of a combination of beta carotene and vitamin A on lung cancer and cardiovascular disease. NEJM 1996; 334:1150–55.

10. Boehm F, Edge R, McGarvey D J, Truscott T G. Beta-carotene with vitamins E and C offers synergistic cell protection against NOx. FEBS Letter 1998; 436:387–89.

11. Paolini M et al. Co-carcinogenic effect of beta-carotene. Nature 1999; 398:760–61.

12. Cassano P, Hu G at FASEB meeting in San Francisco, April 98.

13. Van Poppel G, Goldbohm R A. Epidemiological evidence for beta carotene and cancer prevention. Am J Clin Nutr 1995; 62:1393S–402S.

14. Jumaan A O, Holmberg L, Zack M et al. Beta-carotene intake and risk of postmenopausal breast cancer. Epidemiology 1999; 10:49–53.

15. Presentation by M Stampfer, American Society of Clinical Oncology annual meeting, Denver, 19 May 1997.

16. Acevedo P, Bertram J S. Liarozole potentiates the cancer chemopreventive activity of and the upregulation of gap junction communication and connexin 43 expression by retinoic acid and beta-carotene in 10T1/2 cells. Carcinogenesis 1995; 16:2215–22.

17. Nieper H. Technology, Medicine, and Society. MIT Verlag 1985, 268–69.

18. Santos, M S et al. Beta-carotene-induced enhancement of natural killer cell activity in elderly men: an investigation of the role of cytokines. Am J Clin Nutr 1998; 68:164–70.

19. Canfield L M, Forage J W, Valenzuela J G. Carotenoids as cellular antioxidants. Proceedings of the Society of Experimental Biology and Medicine 1992; 200:260–65.

20. Di Mascio P, Kiaser S, Sies H. Lycopene as the most efficient biological carotenoid singlet oxygen quencher. Arch Biochem Biophys 1989; 274:532–38.

21. Giovannucci E, Ascherio A, Rimm E B, Stampfer M J, et al. Intake of carotenoids and retinol in relation to risk of prostate cancer. J Natl Cancer Institute 1995; 87:1767–76.

22. Presentation by O Kucuk, Karmanos Cancer Institute, American Association for Cancer Research meeting, 12 April 1999.
23. Giovannucci E. Tomatoes, tomato-based products, lycopene, and cancer: review of the epidemiological literature. J Natl Cancer Institute 1999; 91:317–31.
24. Garcia-Closas R, Agudo A, Gonzales C A, Riboli R E. Intake of specific carotenoids and flavonoids and the risk of lung cancer in women in Barcelona, Spain. Nutr Cancer 1998; 32: 154–58.
25. Kohlmeier L, Kark J D et al. Lycopene and myocardial infarction risk in the EURAMIC Study. Am J Epidemiology 1997; 146:618–26.
26. Riso P, Pinder A et al. Does tomato consumption effectively increase the resistance of lymphocyte DNA to oxidative damage? Am J. Clin Nutr 1999; 69:712–18.
27. Christen W G, Glynn R J et al. A prospective study of cigarette smoking and the risk of age-related macular degeneration in men. JAMA 1996; 276:1147–51; Seddon J M, Willett W C et al. A prospective study of cigarette smoking and the risk of age-related macular degeneration in women. JAMA 1996; 276:1141–46.
28. Snodderly, D M. Evidence for protection against age-related macular degeneration by carotenoids and antioxidant vitamins. Am J Clin Nutr 1995; 62S:1448S–61S.
29. Seddon J M, Ajani U A, Perduto R D et al. Dietary carotenoids, vitamins A, C, and E, and advanced age-related macular degeneration. JAMA 1994; 272:1413–20.
30. Sommerburg O et al. Fruits and vegetables that are sources for lutein and zeaxanthin: the macular pigment in human eyes. Brit J Ophthalmology 1998; 83:907–10.
31. Seddon, Ajani, Perduto et al. Dietary carotenoids . . .
32. Stampfer M J, Willett W C. Olestra and the FDA. NEJM 1996; 335:669.

Chapter 11

1. Witte J S et al. Relation of vegetable, fruit, and grain consumption to colorectal adenomatous polyps. Am J Epidemiology 1996; 144:1015–25.
2. Prior R L, Cao G. Antioxidant capacity and polyphenolic components of teas: implications for altering in vivo antioxidant status. Proc Soc Exp Biol Med 1999; 220:255–61.
3. Gao Y T, McLaughlin J K, Blot W J et al. Reduced risk of

esophageal cancer associated with green tea consumption. J Natl Cancer Institute 1994; 85:855–58.

4. Katiyar S K and Mukhtar H. Tea in chemoprevention of cancer: epidemiologic and experimental studies. International J of Oncology 1996; 8:221–38.

5. Ahmad N, Feyes D K et al. Green tea constituent epigallocatechin-3-gallate and induction of apoptosis and cell cycle arrest in human carcinoma cells. J Natl Cancer Institute 1997; 89:1881–86.

6. Presentation by D J Morré and D M Morré, American Society for Cell Biology annual meeting, December 1998.

7. Luo M, Kannar K, Wahlqvist M L, O'Brien R C. Inhibition of LDL oxidation by green tea extract. Lancet 1997; 349:360–61.

8. Sesso, H D et al. Coffee and tea intake and risk of myocardial infarction. Am J Epidemiology 1999; 149:162–67.

9. Keli S O et al. Dietary bioflavonoids, antioxidant vitamins, and incidence of stroke: the Zutphen Study. Archives of Internal Medicine 1996; 156:637–42.

10. Haqqi T M et al. Prevention of collagen-induced arthritis in mice by a polyphenic fraction from green tea. Pro Natl Acad Sci USA 1999; 96:4524–29.

11. Yam T S, Hamilton-Miller J M, Shah S. The effect of a component of tea (Camellia sinensis) on methicillin resistance, PBP2' synthesis, and beta-lactamase production in Staphylococcus aureus. Journal of Antimicrobial Chemotherapy 1998; 42:211–16.

12. Ioky K et al. Antioxidative activity of quercetin and quercetin monoglucosides in solution and phospholipid bilayers. Biochem Biophys Acta 1995; 1234:99–104.

13. Breithaupt-Groegler K, Ling M, Boudoulas H, Betz G G. Protective effect of chronic garlic intake on elastic properties of aorta in the elderly. Circulation 1997; 96:2649–55.

14. Kosceilny J, Kluessendorf D, Latza R et al. The antiatherosclerotic effect of Allium sativum. Atherosclerosis 1999; 144:237–49.

15. Science News 19 April 1997; 151:239.

Chapter 12

1. Barrett-Connor E, Goodman-Gruen D. The epidemiology of DHEAS and cardiovascular disease. Ann NY Acad Sci 1995; 774:259–70.

2. Morales A J, Nolan J J, Nelson J C, Yen S S. Effects of replacement dose of dehydroepiandosterone in men and women of advancing age. J Clin Endocrinology 1994; 78:1360–67.

3. Barrett-Connor E, Khaw K T, Yen S S. A prospective study of dehydroepiandrosterone sulfate, mortality, and cardiovascular disease. NEJM 1986; 315:1519–24.

4. Newcomer, L M, Manson J E, Barbieri R L et al. Dehydroepidandrosterone sulfate and the risk of myocardial infarction in US male physicians: a prospective study. Am J. Epidemiology, 1994; 140:870–75; Herrington D M. Dehydroepiandrosterone and coronary atherosclerosis. Ann NY Acad Sci 1995; 774:271–80.

5. Herrington. Dehydroepiandrosterone and coronary atherosclerosis. Ann NY Acad Sci 1995; 774:271–80.

6. Khorram O, Vu L, and Yen S S. Activation of immune function by dehydroepiandrosterone (DHEA) in age-advanced men. Journal of Gerontology 1997; 52:1–7.

7. Gordon G B, Helzlsouer K J, Comstock G W. Serum levels of dehydroepiandrosterone and its sulfate and the risk of developing bladder cancer. Cancer Res 1991; 51:1366–69; Schwartz A G, Pashko L L. Mechanism of cancer preventive action of DHEA. Ann NY Acad Sci 1995; 774:180–86.

8. Yen S S, Morales A J, Khorram O. Replacement of DHEA in aging men and women. Ann NY Acad Sci 1995; 774:128–42.

9. Flood J F, Morley J E, Roberts E. Memory-enhancing effects in male mice of pregnenolone and steroids metabolically derived from it. Proceedings of Nat Acad Sciences USA 1992; 89:1567–71.

10. Roberts E. Pregnenolone from Selye to Alzheimer and a model of the pregnenolone binding site on the GABA receptor. Biochemical Pharmacology 1995; 49:1–16.

Chapter 13

1, Yesalis C, King D et al. JAMA 1999; 281:2020–28, 2043–44.

2. Barrett-Connor E L. Testosterone and risk factors for cardiovascular disease in men. Diabetes Metab 1995; 21:156–61.

3. Krotkiewski M, Bjorntorp P. The effect of progesterone and of insulin administration on regional adipose tissue cellularity in the rat. Acta Physiol Scand 1976; 96:122–27.

4. Beck P, Eaton R P, Arnett D M et al. Effect of contraceptive

steroids on arginine-stimulated glucagon and insulin secretion in women: I-Lipid physiology. Metabolism 1975; 24:1055–65.

5. Hulley S. Grady D, Bush T et al. Randomized trial of estrogen plus progestin for secondary prevention of coronary heart disease in postmenopausal women: Heart and Estrogen/progestin Replacement Study (HERS) Research Group. JAMA 1998; 280:605–13.

6. Lee J R. Is natural progesterone the missing link in osteoporosis prevention and treatment? Medical Hypotheses 1991; 35:316–18.

7. Agnusdei D, Bufalino L. Efficacy of ipriflavone in established osteoporosis and long-term safety. Calcif Tissue Int 1997; 61: S23–27; Agnusdei D, Crepaldi G, Isaia G et al. A double blind, placebo-controlled trial of ipriflavone for prevention of postmenopausal spinal bone loss. Calcif Tissue Int 1997; 61: 142–47.

8. Rosen T, Johannsson G et al. Consequences of growth hormone deficiency in adults and the benefits and risks of recombinant human growth hormone treatment. A review paper. Horm Res 1995; 43:93–99.

9. Mantzoros C S et al. Insulin resistance: the clinical spectrum. Adv Endocrinol and Metab 1995; 259:1703–05.

10. Rudman D et al. Effect of human growth hormones in men over 60 years old. NEJM 1990; 323:1–6.

11. Fazio S et al. A preliminary study of growth hormone in the treatment of dilated cardiomyopathy. NEJM 1996; 334:809–14.

12. Moses A C. Recombinant human insulin-like growth factor 1 increases insulin sensitivity and improves glycemic control in type II diabetes. Diabetes 1996; 45:91–100.

13. Bennett R M, Clark S C, Walczyk J. A randomized double-blind placebo-controlled study of growth hormone in the treatment of fibromyalgia. Am J Med 1998; 104:227–31.

14. Waters D et al. Recombinant human growth hormone, insulin-like growth factor 1, and combination therapy in AIDS-associated wasting. Ann Intern Med 1996; 125:865–72.

15. Thompson R L. J Clin Endocrinol Metab 1998; 83:M77–84.

16. Yen S S, Morales A J, Khorram O. Replacement of DHEA in aging men and women. Potential remedial effects. Ann NY Acad Sci 1995; 774:128–42.

17. Alba-Roth J, Muller O A, Schopohl J et al. Arginine stimulates growth hormone secretion by suppressing endogenous

somatostatin secretion. J Clin Endocrinol Metab 1988; 67: 1186–89.

18. Borst J E et al. Studies of GH secretogogues in man. J Am Geriatrics Soc 1995; 42:532–34.

19. Corpas E, Blackman M R, Roberson R et al. Oral arginine-lysine does not increase growth hormone or insulin-like growth factor 1 in old men. J Gerontology 1993; 48:M128–33.

20. Welbourne T. Increased plasma bicarbonate and growth hormone after oral glutamine load. Am J Clin Nutr 1995; 61: 1058–61.

21. Rolandi E et al. Changes of pituitary secretion after long-term treatment with Hydergine, in elderly patients. Acta Endocrinologica 983; 102:32–36.

22. Iranmanesh A, Lizarralde B, Veldhuis J D. Age and relative adiposity are specific negative determinants of the frequency and amplitude of growth hormone (GH) secretory bursts and the half-life of endogenous GH in healthy men. J Clin Endocrinol Metab 1991; 73:1081-88.

Chapter 14

1. Castelli. Concerning the possibility of a nutritional . . .

2. Corr L A, Oliver M F. The low fat/low cholesterol diet is ineffective. Eur Heart J 1997; 18:18–22.

3. Ravnskov U. The questionable role of saturated and polyunsaturated fatty acids in cardiovascular disease. J Clin Epidemiol 1998; 51:442–60.

4. Presentation by D L Tirshwell, 24th Annual AHA Conference on Stroke and Cerebral Circulation 10 February 1999.

5. Dreon D M, Fernstrom H A, Williams P T, Krauss R M. A very low-fat diet is not associated with improved lipoprotein profiles in men with a predominance of large, low-density lipoproteins. Am J Clin Nutr 1999; 69:411–18.

6. Bang H O, Dyerberg J, Hjorne N. The composition of food consumed by Greenland Eskimos. Acta Med Scand 1976; 200:69–73.

7. Marchioli R. Lancet 1999; 354:447–55.

8. Burr M I et al. Effects of changes in fat, fish, and fibre intakes on death and myocardial reinfarction: diet and reinfarction trial (DART). Lancet 1989; 2:757–61.

9. Albert C M, Hennekens C H, O'Donnell C J et al. Fish consumption and risk of sudden cardiac death. JAMA 1998; 279: 23–28.

10. Fernandez E, Chatenoud L, La Vecchia C et al. Fish consumption and cancer risk. Am J Clinical Nutr 1999; 70:85–90.

11. Belluzi A, Brignola C, Campieri M et al. Effect of an enteric-coated fish-oil preparation on relapses in Crohn's disease. NEJM 1996; 334:1557–60.

12. Watkin B A, Seifert M F, Allen K G. Importance of dietary fat in modulating PGE2 responses and influence of vitamin E on bone morphometry. Word Rev Nutr Diet 1997; 82:250–59.

13. Stoll A L, Severus W E, Freeman M P et al. Omega 3 fatty acids in bipolar disorder: a preliminary double-blind, placebo-controlled trial. Archives of General Psychiatry 1999; 56:401–12.

14. Zurier R B, Rosetti R G, Jacobson E W et al. Gamma-linolenic acid treatment of rheumatoid arthritis. A randomized, placebo-controlled trial. Arthritis Rheum 1996; 39:1808–17.

15. Hu F B, Stampfer M J, Manson J E et al. Dietary intake of alpha-linolenic acid and risk of fatal ischemic heart disease among women. Am J Clin Nutr 1999; 69:890–97.

16. Hansen J C, Pedersen H S, Mulvad G. Fatty acids and antioxidants in the Inuit diet. Arctic Med Res 1994; 53:4–17.

17. Hu F B, Stampfer M J, Manson J E et al. Frequent nut consumption and risk of coronary heart disease in women: prospective cohort study. BMJ 1998; 317:1341–45.

18. Solfrizzi V, Panza F, Torres F et al. High monounsaturated fatty acids intake protects against age-related cognitive decline. Neurology 1999; 52:1563–69.

19. Willett W C, Stampfer M J, Manson J E et al. Intake of trans fatty acids of risk of coronary heart disease among women. Lancet 1993; 341:581–85.

20. Mann G V. Metabolic consequences of dietary trans fatty acids. Lancet 1994; 343:1268–71.

21. Barnard D E, Sampugna J, Berlin E et al. Dietary trans fatty acids modulate erythrocyte membrane fatty acyl composition and insulin binding in monkeys. J Nutr Biochem 1990; 1:190–95; Kuller L H. Trans fatty acids and dieting [letter]. Lancet 1993; 341:1093–94.

22. Ascherio A, Katan M B, Stampfer M J. Trans fatty acids and coronary heart disease. NEJM 1999; 340:1994–98.

23. Enig M G. Trans Fatty Acids in the Food Supply. Silver Spring, MD: Enig Associates, 1993.

Chapter 15

1. Bernstein J et al. Depression of lymphocyte transformation following oral glucose ingestion. AM J Clin Nutr 1977; 30: 613.

2. Canfield L M, Forage J W, Valanzuela J G. Carotenoids as cellular antioxidants. Proceedings of the Society of Experimental Biology and Medicine 1992; 200:260–65.

3. Santos M S, Meydani S N, Leka L et al. Natural killer cell activity in elderly men is enhanced by beta-carotene supplementation. AM J Clin Nutr 1996; 64:772–77.

4. Chasen-Taber L et al. J Am Coll Nutr 1996; 15:136–43.

5. Bendich A. Food Technology 1987; 41:112–14.

6. Hemila H, Herman Z S. Vitamin C and the common cold: a retrospective analysis of Chalmer's review. J Amer Coll Nutr 1995; 14:116–23.

7. Henson D E, Block G, Levine M. Ascorbic acid: biologic functions and relation to cancer. J Natl Cancer Institute 1991; 83:547–50.

8. Block, G. Vitamin C and reduced mortality. Epidemiology 1992; 3:189–91.

9. Meydani S N, Meydani M, Blumberg J B et al. Vitamin E supplementation and in vivo immune response in healthy elderly subjects: a randomized controlled trial. JAMA 1997; 277:1380–86.

10. Watson R R, Benedict J, Mayberry J C et al. Supplementation of vitamins C and E and cellular immune function in young and aging men. Ann NY Acad Sci 1990; 498:530–33.

11. Ford E S, Sowell A. Serum alpha-tocopherol status in the United States population: findings from the Third National Health and Nutrition Examination Survey. Am J Epidemiology 1999; 150:290–300.

12. Mossad S B, Macknin M L et al. Zinc gluconate lozenges for treating the common cold. Ann Internal Med 1996; 125:81–88.

13. National Center for Health Statistics data from NHANES III.

14. Fortes C et al. The effect of zinc and vitamin A supplementation on immune response in an older population. J Am Geriatrics Soc 1998; 46:19–26.

15. Corti M C et al. Serum iron level, coronary artery disease, and all-cause mortality in older men and women. Am J Cardiology 1997; 79:120–27.

16. Scaglione F, Cattaneo G, Alessandria M, Cogo R. Efficacy and safety of the standardized ginseng extract G 115 for potentiating vaccination against common cold and/or influenza syndrome. Drugs under Experimental and Clinical Research 1996; 22:65–72.

17. See D M, Broumand N, Sahl L, Tilles J G. In vitro effects of echinacea and ginseng on natural killer and antibody-dependent cell cytotoxicity in healthy subjects and chronic fatigue or acquired immunodeficiency syndrome patients. Immunopharmacology 1997; 35:229–35.

18. Song Z et al. Ginseng treatment reduces bacterial load and lung pathology in chronic Pseudomonas aeruginosa pneumonia in rats. Antimicrobial Agents and Chemotherapy 1997; 41:961–64.

19. Zhang et al. Ginseng extract scavenges hydroxyl radical and protects unsaturated fatty acids from decomposition caused by iron-mediated lipid peroxidation. Free Radical Biology and Medicine 1996; 20:145–50.

20. Jensen G L et al. A double-blind, prospective, randomized study of glutamine-enriched compared with standard peptide-based feeding in critically ill patients. Am J Clin Nutr 1996; 64:615–21.

21. Caroleo M, Frasca D, Nistico G et al. Melatonin as immunomodulator in immunodeficient mice. Immunopharmacology 1992; 23:81–89.

Chapter 16

1. Herzenberg M. Scandinavian Journal of Rheumatology 1995; 24:207–11.

2. Lancet 1992; 239:1263–64.

3. Staessen J A, Roels H A, Emelianov D et al. Environmental exposure to cadmium, forearm bone density, and risk of fractures: prospective population study. Lancet 1999; 353:1140–44.

4. Pediatrics 1998; 101:6.

5. Pediatrics 1998; 101:10.

6. Lin J L, Ho H H, Yu C C. Chelation therapy for patients with elevated body lead burden and progressive renal insufficiency. Ann Internal Med 1999; 130:7–13.

7. Rudolph C J, McDonagh E W, Wussow D G. The effect of intravenous ethylene diamine tetraacetic acid (EDTA) upon bone density levels. J Advancement Med 1988; 1:79.

8. Deucher D P. EDTA chelation therapy: an antioxidant strategy. J Advancement Med 1988; 1:182.

9. Kindness G, Frackelton J P. Effect of ethylene diamine tetraacetic acid (EDTA) on platelet aggregation in human blood. J Advancement Med 1989; 2:519.

10. World Health Organization. Environmental Health Criteria for Inorganic Mercury, 118. Geneva: WHO, 1991.

11. Frustaci A, Magnavita N, Chimenti C et al. Marked elevation of myocardial trace elements in idiopathic dilated cardiomyopathy compared with secondary cardiac dysfunction. J Am Coll Cardiology 1999; 33:1578–83.

Chapter 17

1. Grundy S M, Balady G J et al. Primary prevention of coronary heart disease. Circulation 1998; 97:1876–87.

2. Hakim A A, Curb J D et al. Effects of walking on coronary heart disease in elderly men: the Honolulu Heart Program. Circulation 1999; 100:9–13.

3. Ekelund L G et al. Physical fitness as a predictor of cardiovascular mortality in asymptomatic North American men. NEJM 1988; 319:1379–84.

4. Wei M, Gibbons L W, Mitchell T L et al. The association between cardiorespiratory fitness and impaired fasting glucose and type 2 diabetes mellitus in men. Ann Internal Med 1999; 130:89–96.

5. Thune I, Brenn T et al. Physical activity and the risk of breast cancer. NEJM 1997; 336:1269–75; Tang R, Wang J Y, Lo S K, Hsieh L L. Physical activity, water intake and risk of colorectal cancer in Taiwan: a hospital-based case-control study. International Journal of Cancer 1999; 82:484–89.

6. Leveille S G, Guralnik J M et al. Aging successfully until death in old age: opportunities for increasing active life expectancy. Am J Epidemiology 1999; 149:654–64.

7. Ferrucci L, Izmirlian G et al. Smoking, physical activity, and active life expectancy. Am J Epidemiology 1999; 149:645–53.

8. Fiatarone M A, Marks E C et al. High-intensity strength training in nonagenarians: effects on skeletal muscle. JAMA 1990; 263:3029–34.

9. Jette A M et al. Exercise—it's never too late: the strong-for-life program. Am J Public Health 1999; 89:66–72.
10. Hayashi T, Tsumura K, Suematsu C et al. Walking to work and the risk of hypertension in men: the Osaka Health Survey. Ann Internal Med 1999; 130:21–26.
11. Hakim A A, Curb J D, Petrovitch H et al. Effects of walking on coronary heart disease in elderly men: the Honolulu Heart Program. Circulation 1999; 100:9–13.
12. Manson J E, Hu F B et al. A prospective study of walking as compared with vigorous exercise in the prevention of coronary heart disease in women. NEJM 1999; 341:650–58.
13. Kramer A F, Hahn S, Cohen N J et al. Ageing, fitness and neurocognitive function. Nature 1999; 400:418–19.
14. Shore S, Shinkai S et al. Immune responses to training: how critical is training volume? J Sports Med Phys Fitness 1999; 39:1–11.
15. Presentation by J T Venkatramen, 4th International Society for Exercise and Immunology Symposium, May 1999.

Chapter 18

1. Vitek M P, Bhattacharya K, Glendening J M et al. Advanced glycation end products contribute to amyloidosis in Alzheimer disease. Proc Natl Acad Sci USA 1994; 91:4766–70.
2. Ross G W, Petrovitch H et al. Characterization of risk factors for vascular dementia: the Honolulu-Asia Aging Study. Neurology 1999; 53:337–43.
3. Coffey, C E, Saxton J A, Ratcliff G et al. Relation of education to brain size in normal aging: implications for the reserve hypothesis. Neurology 1999; 53:189–96.
4. Bassuk S S, Glass T A, Berkman L F. Social disengagement and incident cognitive decline in community-dwelling elderly persons. Ann Internal Med 1999; 131:165–73.
5. Hopfenmuller W. Proof of the therapeutical effectiveness of a ginkgo biloba special extract. meta-analysis of 11 clinical trials in aged patients with cerebral insufficiency. Arzneim-Forsch 1994; 1005–13; Maurer K. Clinical efficacy of Ginkgo biloba special extract Egb 761 in dementia of the Alzheimer type. J of Psych Research 1997; 31:645–55.
6. Le Bars P L, Katz M M, et al. A placebo-controlled, double-blind, randomized trial of an extract of ginkgo biloba for dementia. JAMA 1997; 278:1327–32.

7. Crook T et al. Effects of phosphatidylserine in age-associated memory impairment. Neurology 1991; 41:644–49.

8. Monteleone P, Beinat L, Tanzillo C et al. Effects of phosphatidyl serine on the neuroendocrine response to physical stress in humans. Neuroendocrinology 1990; 52:243–48.

9. Pettegrew J W et al. Clinical and neurochemical effects of acetyl-l-carnitine in Alzheimer's disease. Neurobiology of Aging 1995; 16:1–4; Salvioli G, Neri M. L-acetylcarnitine treatment of mental decline in the elderly. Drugs in Experimental Clinical Research 1994; 20:169–76.

10. Flood J F, Morley J F, Roberts E. Pregnenolone sulfate enhances post-training memory processes when injected in very low doses into limbic system structures. Proc Natl Acad Sci 1995; 92:10806–10.

11. Ibid.

12. Lindenbaum J, Rosenberg I H, Wilson P W et al. Prevalence of cobalamin deficiency in the Framingham elderly population. Am J Clinical Nutrition 1994; 60:2–11.

13. Clarke R, Smith D, Jobst K A et al. Folate, vitamin B_{12}, and serum total homocysteine levels in confirmed Alzheimer Disease. Arch Neurol 1998; 55:1449–55.

14. Houston D et al. Am J Clinical Nutrition 1999; 69:564–71.

15. Morrison L D, Smith D D, Kish S J. Brain S-adenosylmethionine levels are severely decreased in Alzheimer's disease. Journal of Neurochemistry 1996; 67:1328–31.

Chapter 20

1. Woodward M, Tunstall-Pedoe H. J Epidemiology and Community Health 1999; 53:481–87.

Chapter 21

1. NHANES III survey statistic from CDC's National Center for Health Statistics.

2. National Heart, Lung, and Blood Institute statistics.

3. Cao G, Sofic E, Prior R L. Antioxidant capacity of tea and common vegetables. J Agric Food Chem 1996; 44:3426–31; Wang H, Cao G, Prior RL. Total antioxidant capacity of fruits. J Agric Food Chem 1996; 44:701–05.

4. Steinmetz K A, Potter J D. Vegetables, fruit, and cancer prevention: a review. J Am Diet Assoc 1996; 96:1027–39.

5. Bobak M et al. An ecological study of determinants of coro

nary heart disease rates: a comparison of Czech, Bavarian and Israeli men. Int J Epidemiol 1999; 28:437–44.

6. Cao G, Booth S L, Sadowski J A, Prior R L. Increases in human plasma antioxidant capacity after consumption of controlled diets high in fruit and vegetables. Am J Clin Nutr 1998; 68:1081–87.

7. Cao G, Russel R M, Lischner N, Prior R L. Serum antioxidant capacity is increased by consumption of strawberries, spinach, red wine or vitamin C in elderly women. J Nutr 1998; 128: 2382–90.

Chapter 22

1. Internal Medicine News May 15, 1999, p. 52.

INDEX